"Reading and critiquing scientific articles can be daunting, but this book offers a clear, structured, and comprehensive framework. Dr. Reeves has an extraordinary ability to break down complex concepts and make them accessible, relatable, and enjoyable to learn. This book is an invaluable resource for students."

Nina Heilman, *PhD student in Epidemiology, University of Pittsburgh*

"With the explosion of epidemiologic research over the past decade, learners often struggle to navigate the landscape. Fortunately, Dr. Reeves provides a succinct, disciplined, and fun approach for appraising research so students can quickly evaluate the literature and use it to succeed as scholars and healthcare professionals."

John Norbury, *MD, Associate Professor of Physical Medicine and Rehabilitation at Virginia Commonwealth University and former Inaugural Residency Program Director at Texas Tech University Health Sciences Center*

Making Sense of Epidemiological Research

Using clear language and real-world examples, this accessible textbook provides a concise guide to the understanding and critical evaluation of journal articles in epidemiology.

This book offers a step-by-step process, beginning with how to find epidemiologic studies on a given topic. It then shows readers how to identify and assess the key features of a study's design, the methods of data collection and analysis, the conclusions that can be drawn, and finally the questions that remain. Including a chapter exploring the misuse of artificial intelligence, this complete companion shows students not only how to evaluate individual studies but also to synthesize findings across multiple studies on a single topic, as well as guidance on writing a critique of a given article.

Written by an experienced instructor with over 15 years of experience teaching, and including activities so that readers can practice the skills they learn, this will be essential reading for any student of epidemiology, public health, and medicine.

Katherine W. Reeves is Professor of Epidemiology and Associate Dean of Graduate and Professional Studies, School of Public Health and Health Sciences, University of Massachusetts Amherst, USA.

Making Sense of Epidemiological Research

A Student's Guide

Katherine W. Reeves

Routledge
Taylor & Francis Group

LONDON AND NEW YORK

Designed cover image: Getty

First published 2026
by Routledge
4 Park Square, Milton Park, Abingdon, Oxon, OX14 4RN

and by Routledge
605 Third Avenue, New York, NY 10158

Routledge is an imprint of the Taylor & Francis Group, an informa business

© 2026 Katherine W. Reeves

British Library Cataloguing-in-Publication Data
A catalogue record for this book is available from the British Library

ISBN: 978-1-032-76675-1 (hbk)
ISBN: 978-1-041-06925-6 (pbk)
ISBN: 978-1-003-63789-9 (ebk)

DOI: 10.4324/9781003637899

Typeset in Sabon
by codeMantra

Access the Support Material: www.routledge.com/9781003637899

To my father, Payson R. Whitney, Jr.—my first, and best, editor.

Contents

CONTENTS

Acknowledgments

I am forever indebted to many students, colleagues, and friends for their helpful review and feedback throughout the writing process. There are several individuals who merit special acknowledgment. Isabella Caruso inspired me to take on this project in the first place. Madison Poisson provided honest feedback on early drafts from a student's perspective. Elizabeth Cook and Cassandra Spracklen provided expert evaluation of the entire book. Finally, I thank my husband, Mike, and my children, Ella, Whitney, and Luke, for their unwavering encouragement and support.

List of acronyms and abbreviations

AD	Anti-depressant
AI	Artificial intelligence
ANOVA	Analysis of variance
BDI	Beck Depression Inventory
BMI	Body mass index
BPA	Bisphenol-A
CI	Confidence interval
COI	Conflict of interest
CONSORT	CONsolidated Standards Of Reporting Trials
COVID-19	Coronavirus disease 2019
CV	Coefficient of variation
EQUATOR	Enhancing the quality and transparency of health research
HR	Hazard ratio
ICD	International classification of diseases
IUD	Intrauterine device
JAMA	*Journal of the American Medical Association*
JIF	Journal Impact Factor
JNCI	*Journal of the National Cancer Institute*
LOD	Limit of detection
MESH	Medical subject headings
NEJM	*New England Journal of Medicine*
NHANES	National Health and Nutrition Examination Survey
NSAID	Non-steroidal anti-inflammatory drug
OR	Odds ratio
PFAS	Perfluoroalkyl substances
PRISMA	Preferred Reporting Items of Systematic Reviews and Meta-Analyses

RCT	Randomized controlled trial
RR	Risk ratio
STAR	System for Taking notes on ARticles
STROBE	Strengthening the reporting of observational studies in epidemiology
US	United States

Introduction

We are surrounded by "health" studies, whether we are listening to the news, scanning our social media feeds, or reading medical journals. Especially during the recent COVID-19 pandemic, articles about the effectiveness of social distancing, masking, and vaccines were everywhere. Yet, very often we saw that results of scientific articles were misinterpreted, overstated, or taken out of context. Discussions of the study's potential for bias and error were few and far between. Without clear findings and thoughtful analysis of the studies themselves, the general public, and even some health professionals, became (understandably) mistrustful of the field of epidemiology altogether. This is not a new problem. On the face of it, it can be challenging to understand why one study could report a certain result (eggs are bad for you!), while another study on a similar topic could reach the opposite conclusion (no wait, eggs are good for you!). And when these findings are reduced to a headline or a 30-second soundbite, it is easy to see how people could be misled.

So as budding epidemiologists, researchers, and health professionals, you cannot rely on anyone but yourself for a nuanced discussion and evaluation of the relative strengths and limitations of a health study. It is tempting to read the abstract of a scientific article or a story in the media and think that you know enough to make a conclusion. But you cannot stop there. You need to go right to the primary source and read and critically evaluate the full article yourself. *Reading and critically analyzing scientific articles are the foundation of what epidemiologists do and the foundation of evidence-based medicine.* It is an important skill for medical and public health professionals alike. If you are reading this book, you likely already know this. But, you are probably wondering how to read an epidemiologic article carefully, thoroughly, and critically. Students are often assigned to read these articles, but they are rarely taught how to read them logically and systematically. How do you think through all the different pieces of the study, starting from its purpose and design, to its study population and measurements, to its results and conclusions? That is where this book comes in.

DOI: 10.4324/9781003637899-1

The overall goal of this book is to provide you with an approach that can be used for reading epidemiologic articles. You will learn to apply your knowledge of epidemiologic methods and concepts to critically evaluate a study and come away with an appropriate conclusion based on its strengths and limitations. By the end of this book, you will be able to:

- Apply epidemiologic concepts to read and understand journal articles,
- Critically analyze epidemiologic studies and evaluate their validity based on identified strengths and limitations,
- Synthesize epidemiologic literature on a given topic to identify areas of agreement and disagreement and reach an overall conclusion, and
- Communicate your ideas in writing, using the professional style of epidemiologists.

This is not an epidemiology textbook *per se*. While I will cover epidemiologic methods and concepts (and review the key terms and concepts in Chapter 2), I assume that you have already completed introductory graduate-level courses in epidemiology and biostatistics. If you need additional refresher and/or in-depth discussion and exercises, there are many excellent introductory or intermediate epidemiology texts for you to consult.

Using published epidemiologic articles as examples, this book will provide you with tools for identifying epidemiologic concepts in the real world and for understanding how study methodology impacts what conclusions can be drawn. This book is framed with the key questions you'll need to ask and includes a helpful form for abstracting the key pieces of information—along with your own analysis—as you read a journal article.

Once you have mastered how to read a single article, you will learn how to step back and look at the big picture by comparing and contrasting findings across studies. Being able to synthesize multiple studies on a similar topic is itself a critical skill for epidemiologists and health professionals. Understanding the body of literature as a whole is the underpinning of our work as public health and health professionals, whether you are writing a grant application, deciding whether to recommend a certain screening test or medication to your patients, or selecting an intervention to address a public health concern in your community. Seasoned epidemiologists know that a single study is never definitive. Yet too many faculty assume that the ability to compare and contrast and think broadly about the literature is a skill students will naturally develop just by reading more and more articles, without specific instruction about how to put them all together. Most of us are not born with an innate ability to synthesize findings across epidemiologic studies. But, 16 years of teaching undergraduate and graduate students in public health has shown me that students can develop this skill, provided they have some guidance along the way.

Students often tell me that they feel uncomfortable critiquing published studies. They say to me, "who am I to critique the work of an experienced investigator that was published in a peer-reviewed journal?" You are the perfect person, I tell them. You have the knowledge, and you bring a unique perspective. And I also remind them that there is no such thing as a "perfect" epidemiological study. Humans are not lab rats. We usually cannot choose their exposures for them, nor can we ever fully control the effects of possible confounders in observational studies. Even when we do choose participants' exposure status for them, as in a randomized controlled trial, we cannot fully prevent participants from changing their exposure status or dropping out of the study. All studies have strengths and limitations, and you are well-equipped to identify them. What you need is a system for reading the article itself, a way to make it feel less overwhelming and more informative.

In this book, I will teach you a process for reading and critiquing scientific articles that can be broadly applied to epidemiologic and medical literature, and it even comes along with a handy template for taking notes. By breaking the process down into smaller steps and focusing on key questions that you'll need to ask, critically analyzing scientific articles will be much more manageable (and maybe even fun!).

CHAPTER 1

Why do I need to critically evaluate epidemiologic articles?

You have probably noticed that the final section of nearly every scientific article includes a lengthy discussion of the study's results, how they fit into the broader field, and what they mean for science and public health. So, why can't you just read that and call it a day?

While it may save you some time, if you only read the Discussion section, you are going to miss many important details. For example, if the factor you are most interested in is only a secondary aim of the study, you would find important data within the Results section, but the authors might not go into depth about those findings within the Discussion section. Or, imagine that the authors fail to acknowledge some important issue within their study, such as a 5% response rate, or that they used an insufficient or inappropriate approach to measuring their outcome (think, measuring dementia by self-report). Or, imagine that the authors interpret their findings in a way that is, let's just say, "overly generous." Unfortunately, you don't have to use your imagination—these types of issues are widespread. If you only read the Discussion section, you would miss these really important issues. And you'd be missing an opportunity to exercise your brain and ask questions. And don't we all love to ask questions? That's why we are scientists after all.

As I wrote in the Introduction, reading and critically analyzing scientific articles is the foundation of what epidemiologists do. Before you can design your own study to answer a new research question, you need to understand what is already known. Understanding the strengths and limitations of prior work informs your own work and helps you to move the field forward. If you are writing a thesis proposal or a grant application, you need to distinguish your work from what has already been done. This is impossible to do without a careful and thorough review of the literature on your topic, reading with an eye toward identifying the gaps in current knowledge. For example, is there a segment of the population that has been excluded from prior research? Are prior studies all retrospective? Was the measurement of the main exposure or outcome based on self-report, while an objective assessment is now possible? Being able to

DOI: 10.4324/9781003637899-2

read individual studies, generate a thorough critical analysis, and consider the results along with those from other studies on a given topic is incredibly important. This is how you will generate new ideas. You will need to convince your advisor or funding agencies of the importance of your research question and approach.

At this point, you might be thinking,

> But I'm training to be a physician/nurse/therapist/some other type of health professional. I don't have to write a thesis, and I don't want to write grants and do my own research. Why do I need to know how to read an epidemiologic article?

Well, the ability to critically read and evaluate scientific articles is an essential skill for medical and health professionals too. For example, if you want to make truly evidence-based decisions related to patient care, you need to understand the quality of the evidence and if the findings of the study are relevant to your community. You might need to ask yourself questions like, do the findings from this study apply to my patients? Did they study a population with similar type of disease? Is the population studied fundamentally different than my patient in important ways, for example, sex, race/ethnicity, or access to healthcare?

Regardless of why you are looking at the article, you cannot simply read the Abstract (or the Discussion section) and assume that you have the whole picture. You need to identify the strengths and limitations of all components of the study's methods and think carefully about their potential implications on the study's findings. Are the results an accurate representation of the true relationship between the factors examined within the study population (in epidemiology jargon, is the study "internally valid")? Can the results observed within this study population be applied more broadly to other populations (in epidemiology jargon, is the study "externally valid")? To answer these questions, you will need to not only identify the strengths and limitations of the study but also develop your sense of which are the most likely to impact the results and which are less concerning. Remember: there is no such thing as a perfect study!

Before I go any further, let's spend a moment thinking about the word "critique." Students are often asked to "critique" a study or to "write a critique" of an article. The problem with labeling this activity as "critique" is that it seems to make most of us immediately think negatively about the study. We start reading the article through a lens of "what's wrong?" rather than one of "what's right?" While part of your job will be to identify limitations, it will be just as important to identify strengths. A better term for this activity might be "critical analysis." By "critical," I don't mean only finding fault, but rather I mean engaging in a thoughtful, in-depth analytical process of evaluating the article through consideration of its strengths and limitations. In this sense, we can perform a "critical analysis" or "critique" of an excellent study just as we can for a poorly conducted study.

How do epidemiologic articles get published?

It is helpful to understand how an epidemiologic study ends up as a published article. Typically, a group of scientists work together to write up their study findings into a manuscript. Next, they identify a target journal, perhaps based on the journal's reputation or intended audience, and then they submit their manuscript to the journal for consideration. After some general checks by the journal's staff for whether the article would be appropriate for publication in their journal, the manuscript is sent out for peer review by two or more scientists with relevant expertise. These scientists provide a critical analysis of the article, identify major and minor issues to address, and offer a recommendation to the journal's editor as to whether the manuscript should be accepted in its current form, reconsidered after revisions, or rejected altogether. Most articles will go through at least one round of revisions before being accepted for publication by the editor.

The peer-review process is a hallmark of science. It is an important check to confirm that studies are rigorously conducted and accurately reported, and it serves to improve the quality of published work. Articles published in peer-reviewed journals are generally more reliable than those that are not. But, nothing is perfect, and the peer-review process can miss things too. Remember, it is typically only two or three external reviewers reading the manuscript; depending on their expertise and how carefully they read the article, important issues with the study's design or the way the authors interpret their findings may go undetected. While you should always make sure an article has undergone peer review before citing it, you also need to read it yourself and make your own judgments.

Is this a good journal?

Scientific journals vary widely in their quality and in their selectiveness. There really is a difference between citing an article published in the *Journal of the American Medical Association (JAMA)* and an article published in a very small, niche journal with limited readership that publishes everything submitted to it. One obvious metric to use when evaluating the quality of a journal is whether it uses a peer-review process. But, just because a journal uses a peer-review process to evaluate articles doesn't mean that it is a "good" journal. Acceptance rates for a top-tier peer-reviewed journal may be quite low, while lower-tier peer-reviewed journals may publish nearly all manuscripts submitted for their consideration, even those that have some major issues.

One useful metric for evaluating journal quality is the Journal Impact Factor™ (JIF) published in *Journal Citation Reports*.[1] The JIF is calculated for journals every year. The metric is calculated as a ratio of the number of times the articles published in that journal in the prior 2 years were cited by other articles to the total number of articles published in the journal during that time period. The idea is that the more other scientists cite a specific article in their own work, the more impactful that initial article is. And, the more a journal's articles are cited and viewed as impactful, the higher quality the journal is. For example, *Nature* (one of the most prestigious scientific journals) had an impact factor of 64.8 in 2022, while the *Journal of Cancer Epidemiology* (a newer and lesser-known journal) had an impact factor of 1.8 that year.

Impact factors are an easily accessed metric (just do a Google search of the journal's name followed by "impact factor," and you'll have it in less than a second). Recognize, though, that they do tend to favor journals that publish lots of review articles (because review articles tend to be cited frequently) and those that have a broad audience (because the more scientists read an article, the more likely it is to be cited).

Case in point: the 2022 impact factor for the *Journal of the National Cancer Institute (JNCI)*, a prestigious journal for cancer researchers, was 10.3, while the impact factor for the *New England Journal of Medicine (NEJM)* was 158.5. As a cancer researcher, though, I would greatly prefer to have my work published in *JNCI* because it reaches my intended audience, even though the impact factor for *NEJM* is fifteen times higher.

Impact factors are a helpful piece of information, but they don't tell you the full story. There definitely will be a meaningful difference in quality, for example, between a journal with an impact factor above ten and one with an impact factor below one. Beyond such large numerical differences, qualitative data will be helpful in assessing the journal's quality. I do want to note, however, that excellent articles can be published in lower-impact journals (and vice versa). Pay attention to the journals that your instructors, advisors, and colleagues are reading and citing. Where do the leading investigators in your field prefer to publish? What journals do they view with disdain? Noticing and considering these factors will add useful context to the numerical impact factor.

Are there important conflicts of interest?

Identifying conflicts of interest (COIs) can be difficult. Most reputable peer-reviewed journals now require authors to disclose potential COIs, such as reporting funding sources for the research reported in the article as well as for other research activities. These potential COIs are then printed along with the article, typically at the end before the list of references. It is worth noting that just because an author reports a potential COI, it doesn't necessarily mean that their work is tarnished. An author might appropriately report funding from, say, a pharmaceutical company to independently evaluate the safety profile of a new drug, with the company itself having nothing to do with collecting, analyzing, or interpreting the data. The goal of disclosure is to provide the information and then allow readers to make their own judgments.

This system, however, relies on accurate self-reporting. There are some notable examples of how this system can fall short, and even high-quality journals can have an issue. Case in point: a 2019 study made headlines for finding that red meat did not meaningfully impact the risk of cancer or cancer death, noting any increased risk was very small.[2] This finding ran counter to many years of rigorous science demonstrating an increased risk of cancer and cancer death among individuals consuming high levels of red and processed meats. The new findings were from a systematic review and meta-analysis, which we generally would rate among the highest level of evidence, and the article was published in the *Annals of Internal Medicine*, a very high-quality, peer-reviewed journal (2022 impact factor 39.2).

So, good news for bacon lovers, right? Well, not quite. Almost immediately after publication and the widespread media attention, scientists started questioning the findings.[3] Importantly, they recognized that the senior author failed to disclose a financial relationship with an entity funded by the beef industry, ultimately leading the journal to publish a correction noting this potential conflict of interest.[4] For many readers, it felt unsurprising that investigators funded by the beef industry would come to the conclusion that eating red meat didn't increase the risk of cancer or cancer death. This example underscores the importance of considering financial and non-financial COIs when evaluating a scientific article. This case also emphasizes my point that readers cannot rely on anyone but themselves to thoroughly, and critically, analyze the article. In this case, the media, but also the journal's peer reviewers and editors, got it wrong.

What about publication bias?

The need to grab readers' attention isn't just an issue for the popular media! This can have an impact on scientific journals too, though we give it a much more official-sounding name than "clickbait": publication bias. In short, **publication bias** refers to the higher likelihood of an article being accepted for publication if it finds something interesting. For example, an article that reports eating eggs every day triples the risk of heart attacks would be systematically more likely to be published in a scientific journal than an article that reports eggs have no statistical association with heart attack risk.

Why does this matter? After all, most of us would prefer to read something "interesting," right? The problem is that if studies finding no association are systematically less likely to be published than those reporting a positive or negative association, we end up not realizing that those null studies exist. Even the most rigorous search of the literature would not turn them up if they aren't published in the first place. If you reviewed all the existing literature, you would (incorrectly) conclude that there is consistency in finding a positive (or negative) association. Publication bias can have important implications, for example, if you are trying to make evidence-based decisions about the safety or efficacy of a drug.

Scientists now recognize that publication bias exists and that it can lead to inappropriate conclusions. Awareness of the potential for publication bias is one reason why legislation and policies in the U.S. and other countries now require clinical trials to be registered and to report their results. In the U.S., this is accomplished through registration and reporting at ClinicalTrials.gov, under the direction of the National Institutes of Health. Increasingly, journals are making space for authors to report research studies with null results (albeit often with a very limited word count; e.g., *Cancer Epidemiology, Biomarkers & Prevention* allows up to 4,000 words for a full-length article, yet only 800 words for their option to report null findings in an abbreviated article).[5]

Scientists have developed methods for evaluating whether publication bias is present in the literature on a given topic. One of the most common methods is the funnel plot, which is a graphical presentation of studies' results that can be helpful in detecting publication bias. A funnel plot graphs the studies' estimated measure of association (e.g., odds ratio) versus the sample size (or standard error of the estimated measure of association, which is related to the sample size). The overall effect estimate from a meta-analysis (assumed to be the "true effect") can be plotted as a constant line, around which the other studies are plotted. The idea is that the larger studies will be more precise and their estimates closer together, while the smaller studies will be less precise and so more spread out on the graph—this is what gives the plot its characteristic funnel shape. If the plot is symmetrical around the "true effect" line, then publication bias is unlikely—the symmetry suggests that both positive and negative/null results are being published. However, if the plot is not symmetrical, this can indicate that studies with positive (or negative/null) results, especially smaller studies with lower precision (i.e., wider confidence intervals), are less likely to be published.

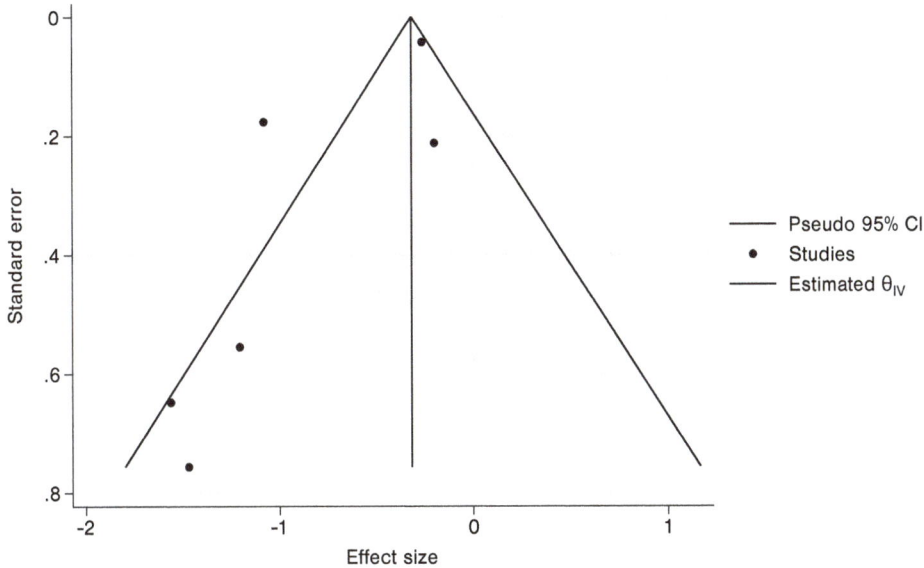

Figure 1.1 Funnel plot of studies evaluating the effectiveness of mask-wearing for the prevention of COVID-19 infection, based upon articles reviewed in Talic et al. (2021).[6]

As an example, Figure 1.1 shows a funnel plot that I created from the results of six articles that were included in a recent meta-analysis to evaluate the effectiveness of masking for the prevention of COVID-19 infection.[6] While the meta-analysis reported a statistically significant 53% decreased risk of COVID-19 associated with mask-wearing, the asymmetry of the funnel plot suggests a possibility of publication bias, with null or negative results perhaps not published. Additionally, the authors of the systematic review and meta-analyses noted significant concerns related to bias in the identified articles and substantial heterogeneity across the study's findings. We also should note, however, that only articles published through June 2021 were included, when the literature was quite new, and that funnel plots are less informative when there are fewer than ten studies included.

Epidemiology and the media: it's complicated

As a scientist, you probably aren't looking to your local news or your social media feed to get your information about issues impacting health. But, you also can't avoid them. Your patients will ask you about them. Your family will ask you about them. Your students will ask you about them. As a public health or health professional, you need to be able to think beyond the headlines and go to the actual source to evaluate their conclusions. Findings are often misrepresented in the media, which underscores the need for all medical and public health professionals to be skilled in reading and critically evaluating scientific articles themselves.

A great example is a study by Kloner et al.[7] that was published early in 2011 and immediately drew significant media attention just before the Super Bowl, the biggest single sporting event in the U.S. each year. Headlines of news articles suggested that a football team losing in the Super Bowl could cause the team's fans to have heart attacks, often accompanied by a picture of overweight football fans screaming for their team, complete with their beer can helmets and team jerseys. But, was there actually evidence that a favorite football team losing in the biggest game of the year could cause heart attacks?

The basic idea of the scientific article was to examine death certificate data from Los Angeles (LA) County for the two weeks following Super Bowls where an LA football team either lost in an epic fourth-quarter meltdown (1980 Rams) or won convincingly (1984 Raiders), comparing the death rates during those 2 weeks to similar weeks of nearby years (other days in January and February in 1980–1984 and 1984–1988, respectively) when an LA team was not in the Super Bowl. There are many problems with the methodology here, but let's just tackle (get it?) three of the biggest ones. First, death certificates are well-known for having systematic inaccuracies, which could lead to bias in the outcome measurement (more to come on that topic in Chapter 7). Second, the study relied on group-level data (in epidemiology jargon, an "ecologic" study), where we have no idea if the individuals who died of heart attacks after the Super Bowl watched, or even cared, about the game. Third, death rates following heart attacks improved markedly throughout the 1980s thanks to advances in medical care. As a result, we would expect to see lower heart attack death rates in 1984 compared to 1980, whether or not the local team won the Super Bowl.

Even if you set aside these issues for a moment and looked carefully at the results tables in the original epidemiology article, you would note that there were actually no significant differences in heart attack deaths following the 1980 Super Bowl; while the numbers show a slight increase following the Super Bowl compared to the control days for both men (0.29 deaths per 100,000 vs 0.25 deaths per 100,000, respectively; p = 0.11) and women (0.26 deaths per 100,000 vs 0.22 deaths per 100,000, respectively; p = 0.06), neither of these differences were statistically significant (meaning the p values—which we will review in Chapter 2—were not ≤0.05). However, many media headlines specifically warned readers of the risk of a heart attack if their favorite team loses the Super Bowl. In fairness, some media articles also included a thoughtful explanation of the main weaknesses of the study. However, I wonder how many people read past the headline or the first provocative sentence.

An illustrative example: antiperspirants and breast cancer

Chances are, you have heard the urban legend about antiperspirants and deodorants causing breast cancer. Any time I have asked classes of undergraduate or graduate students whether they think this link is true or false, a majority vote either true or unsure. Because so many of us use these products on a daily basis, the possibility that they could be putting us at risk for cancer in the future is indeed a scary thought. Rest assured, though, that the prevailing conclusion among scientists is that the evidence does not support a causal connection between the use of antiperspirants or deodorants and the development of breast cancer.

However, if you rely on media reports, you might come to a different understanding about the scientific evidence. A good example is the media coverage that was given to a poor-quality scientific publication on this topic.[8] This study contacted women who had been diagnosed with breast cancer up to 10 years earlier and asked them questions about their use of antiperspirants and deodorants as well as their habits related to underarm shaving. The author concluded that women who reported using these products and shaving most often were diagnosed with breast cancer at earlier ages than those who did not use antiperspirants or deodorants. The ultimate recommendation by the author was that discontinuing the use of these products might lower breast cancer risk.

As with the earlier study connecting Super Bowl defeats to heart attack deaths, there are many issues with the study methodology that we could discuss here. As a prelude to future chapters, Table 1.1 presents the key methodological elements of the

Table 1.1 Summary of key methodological details and their limitations in the McGrath 2003[8] article

Methodological element	Limitations
What study design was used? Unclear	■ Best described as a case-control study because participants were selected based on disease status. However, no controls were enrolled. ■ Lack of a comparison group prevents estimating associations between exposure and outcome.
Who was in the study population? Mailed questionnaires to breast cancer cases diagnosed 1993–2001 and identified via tumor registries at two Chicago hospitals	■ Prevalent (as opposed to incident) cases were included, and only those who were alive in 2002 could be studied. If exposure varied among those who were alive and those who were not, this would bias results. ■ Low response rate (437 participants of 1,344 questionnaires = 32.5%) could bias results if exposure status varies between those who responded and those who did not. At a minimum, it is unlikely that those who responded are representative of all breast cancer cases diagnosed in the study period. ■ Cases diagnosed at the two selected hospitals may not be representative of local or broader populations, which is a major threat to internal validity and also limits external validity.
How was exposure measured? Self-reported on mailed questionnaires; participants instructed to refer to product labels	■ Unclear whether participants were reporting current or past use of antiperspirants/deodorants/shaving; current habits could not impact breast cancer diagnosis. ■ Potential recall bias, if the accuracy of reporting exposure is related to the outcome of age at breast cancer diagnosis. ■ Potential non-differential misclassification, given unclear reporting periods and the need to report age of onset.
How was the outcome measured? Breast cancer diagnoses identified via tumor registry, with age at diagnosis self-reported on mailed questionnaires	■ Cases were prevalent, not incident, which may cause bias as noted above. ■ Age at breast cancer diagnosis is an unusual outcome and is not useful for estimating risk. ■ Unclear whether age at diagnosis and other breast cancer characteristics were obtained from tumor registry data or from self-report, the latter being less valid.

study as well as a brief commentary on the problems with them. A careful and critical reading of the article shows us that: (1) the study could not assess the *risk* of breast cancer (since all women included in the study already had breast cancer), (2) the information collected about antiperspirant/deodorant use and underarm shaving was unlikely to reflect exposure at a time that could have reasonably caused their breast cancer (as breast cancer is believed to take decades to develop before clinical diagnosis and women were likely reporting their current products), and (3) failed to statistically adjust for important, known breast cancer risk factors that could confound an association between antiperspirant/deodorant use and breast cancer (e.g., earlier age at first menstrual period is known to increase breast cancer risk and most women start using antiperspirant/deodorant around this time as well). Overall, the study was poorly designed and executed, and the results are highly affected by bias, error, and confounding. We cannot ignore the many threats to internal validity within the study. When you think carefully about the strengths and limitations related to the study's methodology, it is impossible to support the author's conclusion that these underarm hygiene behaviors cause breast cancer. Yet, the results were incorrectly interpreted, by both the media and the author, to indicate the presence of a causal relationship.

In fact, many scientific studies have explored whether there is an association between antiperspirant use and breast cancer risk. Overwhelmingly, the higher-quality studies to date do not support a causal relationship. Throughout the rest of the book, I will return to this topic frequently for an illustration of how to apply our approach for critically evaluating scientific articles. I will use one of these articles[9] to show how to take notes using a standard template (introduced in Chapter 3) and how to develop those notes into a full-length written critical analysis (covered in Chapter 9). We also will explore this topic as we consider how to synthesize across multiple articles on a given topic. As I develop a critical analysis of this single article, you will see how to put these concepts into practice.

Activities

1. Look up the impact factors for journals in your field of interest. Try to identify at least one journal that has a high impact factor, a medium impact factor, and a low impact factor.
2. For each of the journals you identified, read the publication policies that are posted on their website. Are manuscripts peer-reviewed? Is there a clear policy about disclosure of potential conflicts of interest? What other instructions are given to authors?
3. Identify a health-related news story that is reported by a reputable media outlet. Then, retrieve the scientific article on which the media report was based. How was the scientific article covered in the media report? Did the media report accurately describe the study and its results? Was the media report unbiased? Did the media report sensationalize the scientific findings?

References

1. Journal Citation Reports - Home. Accessed October 27, 2023. https://clarivate.com/products/scientific-and-academic-research/research-analytics-evaluation-and-management-solutions/journal-citation-reports/

2. Han MA, Zeraatkar D, Guyatt GH, et al. Reduction of red and processed meat intake and cancer mortality and incidence: A systematic review and meta-analysis of cohort studies. *Ann Intern Med*. 2019;171(10):711–720. doi:10.7326/M19–0699
3. New "guidelines" say continue red meat consumption habits, but recommendations contradict evidence. *The Nutrition Source*. September 30, 2019. Accessed June 7, 2024. https://nutritionsource.hsph.harvard.edu/2019/09/30/flawed-guidelines-red-processed-meat/
4. Correction: Nutritional recommendations (NutriRECS) on consumption of red and processed meat. *Ann Intern Med*. 2020;172(3):228. doi:10.7326/L19–0822
5. Categories of Articles | Cancer Epidemiology, Biomarkers & Prevention | American Association for Cancer Research. Accessed June 7, 2024. https://aacrjournals.org/cebp/pages/journal-ifora
6. Talic S, Shah S, Wild H, et al. Effectiveness of public health measures in reducing the incidence of covid-19, SARS-CoV-2 transmission, and covid-19 mortality: Systematic review and meta-analysis. *BMJ*. 2021;375:e068302. doi:10.1136/bmj-2021–068302
7. Kloner RA, McDonald SA, Leeka J, Poole WK. Role of age, sex, and race on cardiac and total mortality associated with Super Bowl wins and losses. *Clin Cardiol*. 2011;34(2):102–107. doi:10.1002/clc.20876
8. McGrath KG. An earlier age of breast cancer diagnosis related to more frequent use of antiperspirants/deodorants and underarm shaving. *Eur J Cancer Prev*. 2003;12(6):479–485. doi:10.1097/00008469–200312000-00006
9. Mirick DK, Davis S, Thomas DB. Antiperspirant use and the risk of breast cancer. *J Natl Cancer Inst*. 2002;94(20):1578–1580. doi:10.1093/jnci/94.20.1578

What basic epidemiology and biostatistics concepts should I know?

I have written this textbook assuming that you have successfully completed introductory courses in epidemiology and biostatistics. However, I also understand that: (1) humans can forget things easily, (2) learning often requires repetition, and (3) maybe you didn't quite understand everything the first time around.

In this chapter, I provide a quick-reference guide for you to brush up on what I consider to be the key foundational concepts you will need in order to effectively read and critically analyze epidemiologic studies. We will go more in depth on these concepts as we continue through the textbook. In the following text and tables, I provide you with: (1) a definition of each term, (2) an example, and (3) references to where we'll explore these concepts in depth later in the text.

What are the basic epidemiologic terms?

Most epidemiologic studies are centered around exploring associations between two factors, which are referred to as the exposure and outcome (Table 2.1). The **exposure** is the factor being studied as a potential cause of a disease or condition. Exposures could be any number of demographic, behavioral, medical, social, or other characteristics of individuals or populations. Common exposures include physical measurements (e.g., body weight, blood pressure) and health behaviors (e.g., smoking status, physical activity). The **outcome** is what we call the disease or condition under study. Students sometimes think that the outcome of a study refers to its results, but this is not the case in epidemiology. An outcome could be a disease (e.g., a specific type of cancer), or it could be another characteristic of a population or individual (e.g., a baby's birthweight).

One common point of confusion is that the exposure in one study can be the outcome in another, and vice versa. For example, you could evaluate whether physical activity (as an exposure) is associated with the risk of diabetes (as an outcome). But, you could also evaluate whether diabetes (as an exposure) is associated with the risk of breast cancer (as an outcome). And, you also could evaluate whether breast cancer status (as an exposure) is associated with physical activity (as an outcome). The possibilities are endless! How, then,

DOI: 10.4324/9781003637899-3

Table 2.1 Basic epidemiology terms

Term Chapter	Definition	Examples
Exposure Chapter 6	The factor being studied for a potential association with the outcome of interest	An exposure could be any number of things: a treatment (e.g., a new drug or therapy), a physical measurement (e.g., body weight, blood pressure), a demographic characteristic (e.g., age, race, ethnicity), a behavior (e.g., smoking, physical activity), a social characteristic (e.g., sexual orientation, religion).
Outcome Chapter 7	The disease or condition under study	Could be a diagnosed disease (e.g., specific type of cancer), behavior (e.g., receipt of cancer screening test), or measurable biomarker of disease (e.g., serum triglycerides).
Study population Chapter 5	A group formed by the individual participants for a given study	The entire group of breast cancer cases and matched controls in a case-control study.
Population Chapter 5	A group of individuals who share some common characteristic (e.g., geography, gender, or race/ethnicity) of relevance to the research question	A research study might define its population of interest as all individuals residing in a certain county within a state.
Participant Chapter 5	An individual who contributes data to the research study	A single case of breast cancer in a case-control study.

do you figure out what is the exposure, and what is the outcome in a particular study? Typically, epidemiologists will phrase their research questions and hypothesis statements as looking for associations between [exposure] and [outcome], or asking if [exposure] is predictive of risk of [outcome]. Identifying the exposure and outcome under study is an important first step in reading an epidemiologic article. We will explore additional considerations about the exposure and outcome, and how they are measured in Chapters 6 and 7, respectively.

The **study population** is the group of individuals whose data are gathered and analyzed in the study. We can describe different levels of populations as we select those we will study, starting from the very broad down to the smaller subset of individuals who actually contribute data to the particular analysis; we will explore these selection processes in depth in Chapter 5. For now, you should understand that a **population** is a group of individuals who share some common characteristic (or set of characteristics) that is of relevance to the research question. Populations are often defined by person (e.g., race and ethnicity, gender), place (e.g., country, zip code), and time (e.g., age, year of enrollment). A **participant** is an individual who meets all specific eligibility criteria and contributes data to the research study. As you will see in Chapter 5, who is (and is not) included in the study population and the reasons for their inclusion (or exclusion) will have important effects on the study and what conclusions you can draw from its results.

What are the most common epidemiologic study designs?

We will delve into fine detail on epidemiologic study designs in Chapter 4, but it will be helpful to have some basic definitions and examples in your head even before you read that chapter (Table 2.2). The simplest study design is the **case report** or **case series**.

Table 2.2 Common epidemiologic study designs

Term Chapter	Definition	Example
Case report/ case series Chapter 4	The detailed report of a single or group of cases	Two unusual cases of encephalitis were reported and ultimately led to the recognition of an outbreak of West Nile Virus.[1]
Ecologic Chapter 4	Studies that examine correlations between distributions of exposures and outcomes across populations at the population level	A positive correlation was observed between average dietary fat intake and breast cancer mortality examining population-level estimates from 30 countries.[2]
Cross-sectional Chapter 4	Studies that measure exposure status and outcome status on participants in a defined study population at a single point in time, gather individual-level data, and then estimate associations between exposure prevalence and outcome prevalence within that population	Data from the U.S. National Health and Nutrition Examination Survey (NHANES) demonstrated a U-shaped association between blood levels of perfluoroalkyl substances (PFAS) and depression.[3]
Case-control Chapter 4	Studies that select a group of individuals known to have a particular disease (cases) and a comparable group of individuals known not to have the disease (controls); exposure is then measured in both the cases and in the controls	A study of 362 individuals with pancreatic cancer and 690 randomly selected individuals without pancreatic cancer asked about aspirin use prior to diagnosis and reported that regular, daily aspirin use reduced pancreatic cancer risk.[4]
Prospective cohort Chapter 4	Studies that enroll a group of participants without the outcome of interest and measure exposure status; participants are then followed forward in time to determine who develops the outcome and who does not	A study of 15,792 participants, 1,155 of whom had an ischemic stroke, observed an increased risk of dementia after stroke, over a median 25.5 years of follow-up.[5]
Randomized controlled trial Chapter 4	Studies that assign participants, through a random process, to be exposed or not; participants are then followed forward in time to determine who develops the outcome and who does not	A study of 30,420 participants reported 94.1% efficacy of an mRNA-based vaccine for preventing infection with SARS-CoV-2 compared to placebo.[6]

These are both detailed descriptions of a single case (case report) or group of cases (case series) and often include details about the symptoms, diagnostic journey, and patient characteristics. These reports do not include any comparison group, nor are they framed around a specific hypothesis. Often, case reports/series document new and/or unusual symptoms or conditions. While they cannot provide evidence for causality, they can play highly important roles in describing new conditions and recognizing epidemics in the early stages.

Ecologic studies do explore associations between an exposure and an outcome, but they measure these at the population level instead of the individual level. As a result, they do not offer evidence of causality, but they can be useful for suggesting hypotheses to study in the future. A good example of an ecologic study is a graph that plots each country's gross domestic product (a measure of the value of goods and services produced by the country) against its average lifespan. Such an analysis might suggest a particular relationship between economic advantage and length of life, but because it lacks data on individuals and also does not consider important differences in age, biological sex, and other characteristics that could influence mortality across the countries, it cannot provide causal evidence.

A **cross-sectional study** uses data on individuals to explore associations between exposure and outcome at a particular point in time. For this reason, we sometimes describe cross-sectional studies as a "snapshot." While these studies are often cheaper and faster to conduct than other designs, they measure exposure and outcome at the same time. As a result, we often cannot be certain which came first, an issue that epidemiologists refer to as "temporality." In order for us to say that an exposure *causes* an outcome, we need to know that the exposure came first, so cross-sectional studies provide limited evidence to support causality.

Case-control studies enroll individuals who have a particular outcome (the "cases") and a comparable group of individuals who do not have the outcome (the "controls"). Exposure prior to the outcome occurring (or, during a similar time period for the controls) is measured in both groups, and researchers analyze whether the exposure is more (or less) common among the cases versus the controls. Researchers aim to measure exposure during a time that precedes the outcome, but this is often challenging to say the least. These studies provide better evidence for causality than cross-sectional studies, but their design also opens possibilities for many different forms of bias and error.

A stronger study design is the **prospective cohort study**, in which a group of individuals who do not have the outcome but are considered at risk for the outcome are studied. Each participant's exposure status is measured, and then the participants are followed forward in time to determine who develops the outcome and who does not. Prospective cohort studies provide higher-quality evidence of causality because the study design ensures that exposure precedes the outcome. However, these studies can require huge numbers of participants and extended lengths of time, both of which end up making them quite expensive. We can also describe a **retrospective cohort study**, in which exposure is assessed before the outcome occurs, but the study utilizes records or data collected before the study itself was designed. Retrospective cohort studies are especially common in occupational studies and in studies utilizing electronic health records.

Finally, a **randomized controlled trial** is an experimental design, where a group of participants who do not have the outcome (but are at risk for it) are enrolled, randomly assigned (e.g., by flip of a coin) to have a particular exposure (or, to not have the particular exposure), and then followed forward in time to see who develops the outcome and who does not. This study design is used to test new pharmaceutical treatments, because it provides superb control for bias, error, and confounding. Randomized controlled trials can be used to test other interventions too (e.g., a new program to encourage cancer screening). While these studies provide excellent evidence in support of causality, they are not always feasible to conduct (e.g., we could not randomly assign participants to smoke tobacco, because of the overwhelming evidence that this is likely harmful to their health).

What are the basic terms for measuring exposures, outcomes, and associations?

Now that we know about our most common study designs and can identify their key ingredients (i.e., exposure, outcome, study population), we need to review some terms related to the measurement of various factors and the associations between them (Table 2.3). First, **incidence** is the occurrence of *new* cases of the outcome within a defined population. We can compare this to **prevalence**, which is a measure of *existing* cases of the outcome in a defined population. Sometimes we also use prevalence to describe the distribution of an exposure in a population (e.g., the prevalence of obesity among U.S. adults). Interestingly, prevalence and incidence are mathematically related to one another: *Prevalence = Incidence × Duration*. As the incidence of a disease increases and its duration in the affected individual increases, the prevalence of that disease also increases. The duration of a disease or condition is impacted by its ability to be treated and/or cured, as well as its fatality. For example, as better treatment for breast cancer has lengthened the duration that people can live with the disease (duration) and improved screening tests have identified more new cases of breast cancer (incidence), the number of people living with breast cancer also has increased (prevalence).

When describing incident cases of an outcome, we can also measure how often they occur and how fast they occur in the population. The **risk (or cumulative incidence)** is defined as how often the outcome occurs in a specific population over a specific period of time. The **rate** is defined as how fast new cases are occurring within a specific population.

As an example, we can consider various statistics measuring the diagnosis of melanoma (a highly invasive form of skin cancer) in the U.S. In 2024, it was estimated that 100,640 incident cases of melanoma would be diagnosed in the U.S. These incident cases are in addition to the approximately 1,449,916 prevalent cases of melanoma among U.S. adults. The lifetime risk of melanoma for U.S. adults was 2.1% in 2018–2021, with new melanoma cases being diagnosed at a rate of 21.2 per 100,000 adults per year.[11]

We can use measures of association to quantify relationships between the occurrence of exposure and outcome within a population. A **risk ratio (RR)**, which sometimes is referred to as the **relative risk** or estimated using a **hazard ratio**, is the mathematical ratio of the incidence of the outcome among those who are exposed to the incidence of the outcome among those who are not exposed. Similarly, a **rate ratio** is the mathematical ratio of the incidence **rate** among those who are exposed to those who are not exposed.

Table 2.3 Key terms for measuring exposures, outcomes, and associations

Term	Definition	Example
Incidence	The occurrence of new cases of outcome, or new instances of exposure, in the population	Approximately 152,810 new cases of colorectal cancer will be diagnosed among U.S. adults in 2024.[7]
Prevalence	The number of existing cases of outcome in the population	Approximately 1,392,445 U.S. adults are living with colorectal cancer, as of 2021.[7]
Risk (or cumulative incidence)	How often an outcome occurs in a defined group of people in a defined period of time	The lifetime risk of colorectal cancer is 4.0% for U.S. adults.[7]
Rate	How fast new cases of the outcome occur in a population	New colorectal cancer cases are diagnosed among U.S. adults at a rate of 36.5 per 100,000 annually.[7]
Risk ratio	A ratio comparing the risk of outcome in the exposed group to the risk of outcome in an unexposed group	A prospective cohort study evaluating coffee as a risk factor for colorectal cancer reported a risk ratio of 1.15, indicating a slight increased risk of colorectal cancer comparing coffee drinkers to nondrinkers.[8]
Rate ratio	A ratio comparing the rate of outcome in the exposed group to the rate of outcome in the unexposed group	A prospective cohort study evaluating a blood biomarker of whole-grain rye and wheat consumption in relation to distal colorectal cancer risk reported an incidence rate ratio of 0.48 comparing those in the highest vs lowest quartile of the biomarker, suggesting that intake of whole-grain rye and wheat may reduce incidence of distal colorectal cancer.[9]
Odds ratio	A ratio of the odds of exposure among those who have the outcome to the odds of exposure among those who do not have the outcome	A case-control study evaluating a specific dietary pattern in relation to colorectal cancer reported an odds ratio of 0.77 for those in the highest tertile vs lowest tertile of adherence to the dietary pattern, indicating following the particular dietary pattern reduced risk of colorectal cancer.[10]

Because case-control studies select participants who are already known to have (or not have) the outcome, we cannot directly measure the risk of the outcome, and thus we cannot directly calculate the RR either. Instead, we can calculate the **odds ratio (OR)**, which is the mathematical ratio of the odds of exposure among those with the outcome to the odds of exposure among those without the outcome. The **odds** are calculated as the probability of having the exposure divided by the probability of not having the exposure; odds are separately calculated among those with and without the outcome.

Regardless of whether we have calculated an RR, a hazards ratio, a rate ratio, or an OR, we interpret the measure in relation to a value of 1. When the risks (or hazards, rates, or odds) are the same in both groups, the ratio will equal 1, and we can say that there is no association between exposure and outcome. When the ratio's value is greater than 1, we can say that the exposure is *positively* associated with the outcome, and when the ratio's value is less than 1, we can say that the exposure is *negatively* associated with the outcome.

What terms describe the performance of measurement tools?

Validity refers to how well an observation aligns with the truth. In other words, we describe a test or experiment as valid when its result is correct. We can describe a measurement approach or tool as valid when the measured value equals the true value (Table 2.4).

Table 2.4 Terms relating to the performance of measurement tools

Term Chapter	Definition	Example
Validity Chapter 6	The ability of a test/instrument to measure the true value	A screening questionnaire for depression can be compared to a gold-standard diagnostic interview to determine its validity.
Reliability Chapter 6	The ability of a test/instrument to produce the same result upon repeated assessments	A screening questionnaire for depression can be given to the same participant at multiple times to assess its reliability.
Accuracy Chapter 6	The combination of the reliability and the validity of the measurement tool	A highly accurate screening questionnaire for depression would have high agreement with the gold standard diagnostic interview and also give the same measurement upon repeated assessment.
Sensitivity Chapter 7	The ability of a test to accurately identify true cases of disease, compared to a gold standard; calculated as the number of true positives (TP) divided by the total number of people with disease (TP + FN) and expressed as a percentage	The sensitivity of an at-home test for SARS-CoV-2 was 50%, meaning that approximately half of true COVID-19 cases were identified using the test.[12]
Specificity Chapter 7	The ability of a test to accurately identify individuals without disease compared to a gold standard; calculated as the number of true negative (TN) results divided by the total number of individuals without disease (TN + FP) and expressed as a percentage	The sensitivity of an at-home test for SARS-CoV-2 was 97%, meaning that nearly all individuals without SARS-CoV-2 infection were identified as negative by the at-home test.[12]

We can also describe the **reliability** of a measurement, which refers to the ability of a measurement approach or instrument to give the same result upon repeated administration. In other words, a fully reliable measurement tool will give the same answer every time. The **accuracy** of a measurement tool reflects both its reliability and validity; in other words, a highly accurate measurement tool will give the correct results (high validity) every time it is repeated (high reliability).

Often when we talk about tests to identify cases of a disease or condition, we calculate their sensitivity and specificity. **Sensitivity** is the ability of a test to accurately identify true cases of disease compared to a gold standard. We can calculate sensitivity by dividing the number of true positive cases (i.e., people who are known to have the outcome and have a positive result on the test) by the total number of people who are known to have the outcome. **Specificity** is the ability of a test to accurately identify individuals who do not have the disease or outcome compared to a gold standard. We also can use these statistics to evaluate the accuracy of exposure measurements. In this setting, sensitivity would describe the measurement tool's ability to identify truly exposed individuals and specificity would describe its ability to identify truly unexposed individuals.

What terms describe the validity of a study's results?

In epidemiology, we describe a study to have **internal validity** when its results are an accurate representation of the true relationship between the exposure and outcome within the study population. A study has **external validity** when its results are applicable to other populations beyond the study population. Often, the term **generalizability** is used as a synonym for external validity (Table 2.5).

Table 2.5 Terms describing the validity of a study's result

Term	Definition	Example
Internal validity	The extent to which the study's results are an accurate representation of the true relationship between the factors examined within the study population	A rigorous randomized controlled trial evaluating a new treatment for heart disease had very low possibility of bias, error, and confounding and thus was judged to have excellent internal validity.
External validity	The extent to which the study's results may be applied to populations beyond the study population; often referred to as "generalizability"	Because the randomized controlled trial of the new heart disease treatment had excellent internal validity, and because the new treatment was not anticipated to have a different effect across population characteristics, the study was judged to have excellent external validity.

What are threats to validity?

Epidemiologists often identify **threats to validity** as factors that reduce the ability of the study to observe the correct association between exposure and outcome; common threats to validity include bias, confounding, and random error (Table 2.6).

Let's start with the term we all probably understand the best: error. Put simply, **error** occurs when there is a difference between a measured value and the true value. Error is part of every measurement we take. It can occur due to imprecision in the measurement

Table 2.6 Terms related to threats to validity

Term Chapters	Definition	Example
Threats to validity	A general term for bias, error, and/or confounding that may impact the internal validity of a study	The goal of a critical analysis of an epidemiologic study is to identify and evaluate all possible threats to validity and use that analysis to make an appropriate conclusion.
Error/ misclassification *Chapters 6 and 7*	A difference between the measured value and the true value	An uncalibrated scale adds 5 pounds to the true body weight.
Non-differential misclassification *Chapters 6 and 7*	Error in a measurement that equally affects groups defined by exposure or outcome	An uncalibrated scale is used on a random selection of study participants.
Differential misclassification *Chapters 6 and 7*	Error in a measurement that varies across groups defined by exposure or outcome	An uncalibrated scale is used only for cases in a case-control study.
Bias *Chapters 5, 6, and 7*	A systematic error	Because the uncalibrated scale is systematically used only on cases, we could describe the measurement of weight in the case-control study as biased.
Information (or measurement) bias *Chapters 6 and 7*	An umbrella term for a systematic error that affects the measurement of exposure, outcome, or other factors under study	There is information bias in the case-control study that uses an uncalibrated scale only for the cases.
Selection bias *Chapter 5*	An umbrella term for a systematic error that arises when the probability of inclusion in the study population is affected by exposure and outcome	A selection bias exists in a study that enrolls 100% of exposed cases but only 50% of unexposed cases.
Confounding *Chapter 8*	A third factor that is non-causally associated with exposure and causally associated with the outcome and thus affects the apparent association between the exposure and outcome being studied	Coffee drinkers are more likely to smoke cigarettes than to be nonsmokers, thus smoking status would confound an apparent association between coffee and lung cancer.

tool, mistakes on the part of the reader, or just random variation. In epidemiology, we often refer to measurement error as **misclassification**. When the measurement error affects all groups, we say that there is **non-differential misclassification**. However, when the level of error is different across (or, affects only some) groups defined by exposure (for classification of the outcome) or by outcome (for classification of the exposure), we say that there is **differential misclassification**. These concepts often are difficult for students to grasp. We will delve into far greater detail on misclassification and how it affects internal validity as we explore exposure assessment (Chapter 6) and outcome assessment (Chapter 7).

Bias is a systematic error that occurs in a study, and it presents a serious threat to internal validity. Epidemiologists divide bias into two categories: selection bias and information bias. **Selection bias** is an umbrella term for a systematic error that arises when the probability of inclusion in the study population is affected by exposure and outcome. Imagine a case-control study to evaluate whether smoking is associated with heart attacks that excludes individuals who had fatal heart attacks. If the prevalence of smoking exposure differs between those with fatal heart attacks and those who survived their heart attack, then a selection bias has occurred that will systematically alter (i.e., bias) the observed association between smoking and heart attack risk. **Information bias** (sometimes referred to as **measurement bias**) is an umbrella term for systematic errors that affect the measurement of exposure, outcome, or other factors under study. Imagine that in the same case-control study of smoking and heart attacks, the cases are asked about their smoking exposure through an in-depth interview that collects data on the age they first smoked, how many packs per day they smoked, and how many years they smoked, while the controls are simply asked, "have you every smoked?" The validity of the smoking data would be quite different using these two approaches. Because the level of misclassification (i.e., error) differs between cases and controls, we would call this differential misclassification, which is another way of saying measurement bias.

Finally, we need to talk about **confounding**, which is a phenomenon that occurs when a third factor that is causally related to the outcome and also non-causally related to the exposure affects the observed association between the exposure and outcome. Going back to our smoking and heart attacks example, we know that increasing age causally increases the risk of heart attack. And, we also know that patterns of smoking behavior differ across age groups, yet not because age *causes* someone to smoke or not smoke. Age is sometimes described as the "universal confounder" because it has such a strong potential to confound a broad set of potential exposure–outcome associations.

What statistical terms should I know?

Let's review some of the most important concepts in biostatistics that you should know to fully understand and interpret the results of epidemiologic studies (Table 2.7). The goal here is not to provide in-depth discussion and theory. If any of these topics are new to you, or if you feel like you need more than just a basic refresher, you should spend some time reviewing your favorite introductory biostatistics textbook (or, review my favorite biostatistics textbook[1]).

Hypothesis testing

All analytic epidemiologic studies should start with a clearly stated hypothesis. Typically, these hypotheses will be framed in terms of the exposure–outcome relationship under

Table 2.7 Basic statistical analysis terms (see Chapter 8 for detailed discussion)

Term	Definition	Example
Null hypothesis	Statement that there is not an association, difference, or effect	There is no association between smoking and lung cancer.
Alternative hypothesis	Statement that there is an association, difference, or effect	There is an association between smoking and lung cancer.
Type I error (α)	The probability of rejecting the null hypothesis given that the null hypothesis is true	The null hypothesis was tested with two-sided $\alpha = 0.05$, meaning there is a 5% chance of incorrectly rejecting the null hypothesis.
Type II error (β)	Probability of failing to reject the null hypothesis given that the null hypothesis is false	The null hypothesis was tested with $\beta = 0.20$, meaning there is a 20% chance of incorrectly failing to reject the null hypothesis.
Statistical power	The ability to detect that an association exists, given that there is truly an association between the variables under study	Because the study had only 50% statistical power, the validity of its observed null association was questioned.
P value	Probability of obtaining a result as or more extreme than the result that was obtained, under the assumption that the null hypothesis is correct	The statistical test indicated a P value of 0.01, indicating a 1% chance of observing that result if the null hypothesis was true.
Confidence interval (CI)	A range of possible values for the result, with a specified degree of confidence. The degree of confidence is directly related to the Type I error rate: X% *confidence* = $(1-\alpha) \times 100\%$.	The odds ratio had a 95% confidence interval that excludes 1, indicating that there was a statistically significant association between exposure and outcome (e.g., OR = 1.5, 95% CI 1.3–1.8).

study. Statistical tests specify a **null hypothesis,** which is a statement that there *is not* an association (or effect, or difference) between the factors under study, and an **alternative hypothesis,** which is a statement that there *is* an association (or effect, or difference) between the factors under study. For example, in our study of smoking and heart attacks, the null hypothesis would be that there is no association between smoking behavior and risk of heart attack (i.e., OR = 1), while the alternative hypothesis would be that smoking behavior is associated with the risk of heart attack (i.e., OR ≠ 1).

You might be wondering why I didn't say that smoking behavior is *positively* associated with the risk of heart attack. When we specify a certain direction of effect, either positive or negative, we are specifying a one-sided hypothesis. Conversely, when we simply state that there is an association (or effect, or difference) without specifying a direction, we have made a **two-sided hypothesis.** Most of the time, epidemiologists specify two-sided hypotheses because we want to leave open the possibility for positive or negative associations. Of course, researchers likely have a particular direction of effect in mind (e.g., smoking increases the risk of heart attack), but they usually

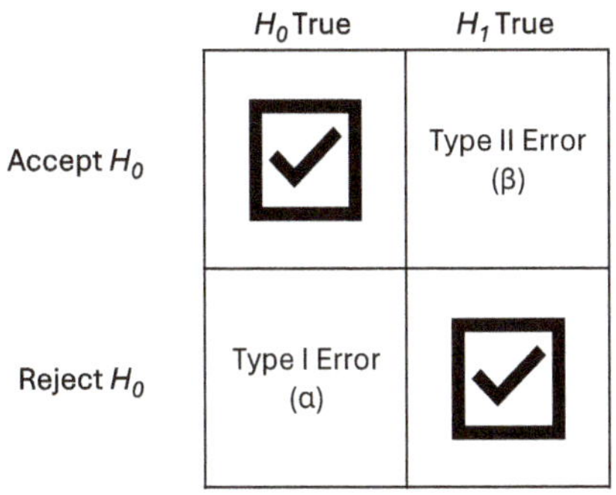

Figure 2.1 Two possible errors can be made in any hypothesis test: (1) Type I error (α), where the null hypothesis is rejected, when in reality it is true, and (2) Type II error (β), where the null hypothesis is accepted, when in reality it is false.

don't set up their statistical testing this way. Sometimes **one-sided hypotheses** are used, though, where a particular direction of effect is specified. For example, in randomized controlled trials to compare a new drug (X) to an existing treatment (A), we might only care about demonstrating that the new drug is better, so we would frame our alternative hypothesis as drug X will increase disease survival compared to drug A.

When we think about statistically testing our hypotheses, we can make two different kinds of errors (Figure 2.1). **Type I error (α)** is when the null hypothesis is rejected by the statistical test even though the null hypothesis is true. For example, we would be making a Type I error if we conclude that there is an association between smoking and heart attacks when there truly is no association between these two factors. Conventionally, we conduct a statistical test of our alternative hypothesis against the null hypothesis, concluding that we reject the null hypothesis based on a predetermined Type I error rate, usually two-sided $\alpha = 0.05$. **Type II error (β)** is when the null hypothesis is *not* rejected even though it actually is false. For example, we would be making a Type II error if we conclude that there is no association between smoking and heart attacks when there actually is an association between these two factors. Because we are more accepting of Type II error than Type I error, we conventionally set the Type II error rate higher than we set the Type I error rate in our statistical tests ($\alpha = 0.05$, $\beta = 0.20$).

P values and confidence intervals

My guess is that P values and confidence intervals (CIs) are the most used, but least understood, concepts in biostatistics. Students often memorize that when $P \leq 0.05$ they reject the null hypothesis, yet students fail to understand the reasoning behind this "rule" or how P values relate to CIs. Understanding what P values and CIs really mean, and how they relate to one another, is crucial for understanding hypothesis testing. By extension, this is crucial for being able to appropriately interpret the results reported in epidemiologic articles.

First, let's define what a P value is. Simply put, a P value is the probability of obtaining a result as extreme or more extreme than the result that was obtained, under the assumption that the null hypothesis is correct. In most cases, we assume that the range of possible values for the association is normally distributed. The null hypothesis value is set at 0 on the standard normal curve (Figure 2.2). The area under the standard normal curve reflects probabilities.

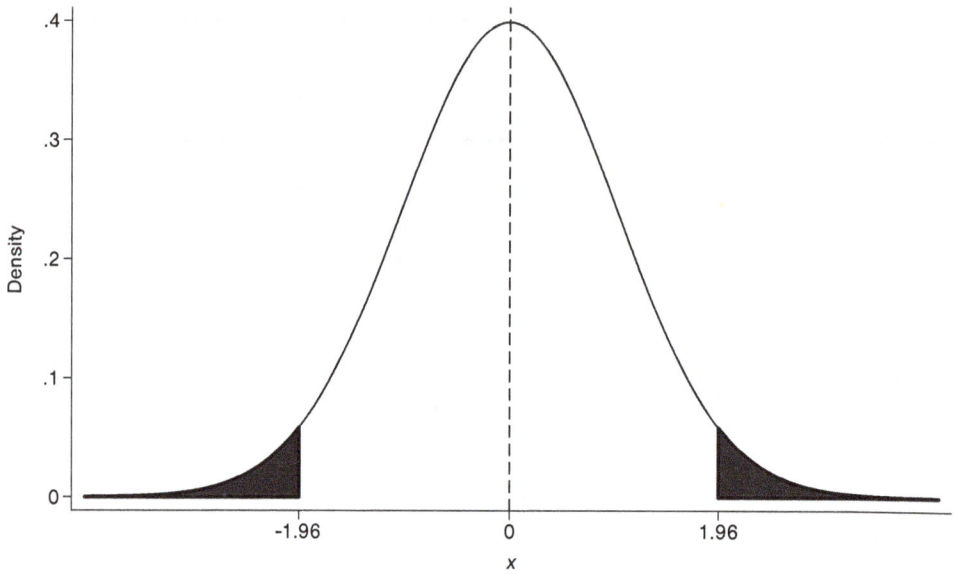

Figure 2.2 The standard normal curve has a mean of 0 and standard deviation of 1. The area under the curve reflects probabilities, with 95% of the area under the curve between –1.96 and +1.96. The area left in the tails of the curves is 2.5% to the left of –1.96 and 2.5% to the right of 1.96. This aligns with a two-sided hypothesis test at $\alpha = 0.05$. When we calculate $P \leq 0.05$, the interpretation is that there is $\leq 5\%$ chance of obtaining a result as or more extreme if the null hypothesis is correct.

To find the probability of obtaining a specific result under the null hypothesis, we find the value of the calculated test statistic on the standard normal curve and calculate the area under the curve to its right (for a positive standardized value) or its left (for a negative standardized value); this is often referred to as the area left in the "tails." For two-sided tests, we sum the areas in both tails to get the P value. Note that we can extend this idea to distributions other than the standard normal (e.g., chi-square distribution), but we will focus on the standard normal distribution here for simplicity. The basic idea is the same: the P value is calculated as the area under the curve in the tail(s).

As an example, let's imagine that we've calculated an OR of 1.50 for our case-control study, and we now want to know if this is statistically different from OR = 1. When we map our effect estimate (OR = 1.50) to the probability distribution curve, we find that there is 4% of the total area under the curve remaining in the two tails; our P value is equal to 0.04. We then can state that there is a 4% probability that we would obtain a result of this magnitude or greater by chance alone, and we conclude that the result is statistically significant at the two-sided $\alpha = 0.05$ level.

CIs are directly related to P values. CIs give a range of possible values for the result, with a specified degree of confidence. The degree of confidence is directly related to the Type I error rate: X% confidence = $(1-\alpha) \times 100\%$. Back to our earlier example, imagine that we calculated a 95% CI of 1.3–1.8 for the estimated OR = 1.5. We would then say that we are 95% confident that the interval from 1.3 to 1.8 includes the true OR. Because the 95% CI excludes 1, we would describe this result as statistically significant with two-sided $\alpha = 0.05$.

While P ≤ 0.05 is commonly used to indicate "statistical significance," the choice of 5% as the chance at which we conclude that the null hypothesis should be rejected is somewhat arbitrary. Why not choose 6%, or 4%? Reliance on P values can lead to binary thinking, where a test result indicates only that the null hypothesis is either true or false. Epidemiologists tend to prefer CIs because they give more information than a P value alone. The CIs give a sense of the direction of the association, even if the result isn't statistically significant. Imagine that our study instead obtained this result: OR = 1.5 (95% CI 0.9–2.3). Because the 95% CI includes the value of 1, this result would not be statistically significant at the two-sided α = 0.05 level. We would correctly conclude that there is not a "statistically significant" association between exposure and outcome. However, the lower limit of the CI is very close to 1, and the upper limit is above 2; this range indicates that it is more likely that there is a positive association than it is that there is a negative association. Using the information from the CI, we could rightly conclude that while the result is not statistically significant, it does suggest a positive association. Importantly, low statistical power might be to blame for the inability to reject the null hypothesis here, so let's consider that topic next.

Statistical power

Statistical power is the ability to detect that an association exists (i.e., to reject the null hypothesis), given that there is truly an association between the variables under study (i.e., given that the null hypothesis is false). Power is directly related to Type II error: Power = $(1 - β) \times 100\%$. Because we conventionally set our Type II error rate at β = 0.20, we conventionally view statistical power of ≥80% as acceptable for testing our null hypothesis.

Statistical power calculations require the use of equations that take into account the desired Type I error rate (conventionally set at α = 0.05), the parameter to be estimated (e.g., difference in means, OR), the sample size, and the expected variability in the measurement among the sample population. Different statistical approaches require slightly different equations for calculating power (i.e., the equation for calculating power when performing a two-sample t-test is different from the equation for calculating power when performing a logistic regression). The equations can get complicated quickly, and most researchers will use statistical analysis software to perform them.

Generally speaking, statistical power increases as (Table 2.8):

- The sample size increases (i.e., larger studies have more power).
- The Type I error rate (α) increases (i.e., making it more likely to reject the null hypothesis increases power).
- The value specified by the alternative hypothesis gets farther away from the null hypothesis (i.e., all other things being equal, there will be greater power to detect an OR of 3.0 as statistically significant than to detect an OR of 1.3 as statistically significant).
- The variability of the parameter within the population decreases (i.e., as the standard deviation of the parameter gets smaller, the statistical power gets larger).
- The variable is scaled continuously as opposed to categorically (e.g., an analysis classifying participants' age to the tenths place, such as 40.8 years, will have more power than the same analysis classifying participants' age into 5-year age groups).

Table 2.8 Statistical power is determined by a number of parameters, including sample size, Type I error rate, alternative hypothesis, and the variability of the parameter. In this example, estimated statistical power for a two-sample t test to compare mean systolic blood pressure between two equally sized groups of adults is shown. Changing the value of one of these parameters, while keeping all the others constant, affects the available statistical power (calculated using Stata v18.0, StataCorp, College Station, TX

Sample size	Type I error rate (α)	Difference in group means	Standard deviation	Calculated statistical power
Original parameter values				
100	0.05	10 mmHg	20	69%
Scenario 1: increase sample size				
200	0.05	10 mmHg	20	**94%**
Scenario 2: increase Type I error				
100	**0.10**	10 mmHg	20	**80%**
Scenario 3: increase mean difference specified as alternative hypothesis				
100	0.05	**20 mmHg**	20	**98%**
Scenario 4: decrease variability of parameter of interest				
100	0.05	10 mmHg	**15**	**91%**

Note: Bold is used to indicate/highlight parameters that have changed in each scenario. Italics is used to separate out each scenario, where a single paramater value is changed from their original values.

Activities

A group of researchers wanted to test the hypothesis that cocaine use increases the risk of having a fatal motor vehicle accident. They identified 200 people who died from a car accident in the prior year by consulting emergency department records at the local hospital. To measure cocaine use in these fatalities, they contacted their next-of-kin and asked, "Did [person's name] use cocaine?" As a comparison group, they asked the first 200 people whom they encountered at the hospital cafeteria, "Do you use cocaine?" They calculated an OR = 1.25 (95% CI 0.85–1.65) for the association between cocaine use and fatal motor vehicle accidents.

1. What type of study design is this?
2. Based on the reported odds ratio and 95% confidence interval, what is the relationship between cocaine use and fatal motor vehicle accident?
3. What problems, if any, do you notice about how the study participants were selected? Describe why these are problems and how they might have affected the study results.
4. What problems, if any, do you notice about how exposure and outcome were measured? Describe why these are problems and how they might have affected the study results.
5. Based on your answers to #3 and #4, do you think this study's results accurately reflect the true relationship between cocaine and fatal motor vehicle accident? Why or why not?

References

1. Outbreak of West Nile-Like Viral Encephalitis -- New York, 1999. Accessed January 9, 2024. https://www.cdc.gov/mmwr/preview/mmwrhtml/mm4838a1.htm
2. Sasaki S, Horacsek M, Kesteloot H. An ecological study of the relationship between dietary fat intake and breast cancer mortality. *Prev Med*. 1993;22(2):187–202. doi:10.1006/pmed. 1993.1016
3. Yi W, Xuan L, Zakaly HMH, et al. Association between per- and polyfluoroalkyl substances (PFAS) and depression in U.S. adults: A cross-sectional study of NHANES from 2005 to 2018. *Environ Res*. 2023;238(Pt 2):117188. doi:10.1016/j.envres.2023.117188
4. Streicher SA, Yu H, Lu L, Kidd MS, Risch HA. Case-control study of aspirin use and risk of pancreatic cancer. *Cancer Epidemiol Biomark Prev Publ*. 2014;23(7):1254–1263. doi:10.1158/1055–9965.EPI-13–1284
5. Koton S, Pike JR, Johansen M, et al. Association of ischemic stroke incidence, severity, and recurrence with dementia in the Atherosclerosis risk in communities cohort study. *JAMA Neurol*. 2022;79(3):271–280. doi:10.1001/jamaneurol.2021.5080
6. Baden LR, El Sahly HM, Essink B, et al. Efficacy and safety of the mRNA-1273 SARS-CoV-2 vaccine. *N Engl J Med*. 2021;384(5):403–416. doi:10.1056/NEJMoa2035389
7. Cancer of the Colon and Rectum - Cancer Stat Facts. SEER. Accessed July 9, 2024. https://seer.cancer.gov/statfacts/html/colorect.html
8. Groessl EJ, Allison MA, Larson JC, et al. Coffee consumption and the incidence of colorectal cancer in women. *J Cancer Epidemiol*. 2016;2016:6918431. doi:10.1155/2016/6918431
9. Kyrø C, Olsen A, Landberg R, et al. Plasma alkylresorcinols, biomarkers of whole-grain wheat and rye intake, and incidence of colorectal cancer. *J Natl Cancer Inst*. 2014;106(1):djt352. doi:10.1093/jnci/djt352
10. Natale A, Turati F, Taborelli M, et al. Diabetes risk reduction diet and colorectal cancer risk. *Cancer Epidemiol Biomark Prev*. 2024;33(5):731–738. doi:10.1158/1055–9965.EPI-23–1400
11. Melanoma of the Skin - Cancer Stat Facts. SEER. Accessed July 2, 2024. https://seer.cancer.gov/statfacts/html/melan.html
12. Chu VT, Schwartz NG, Donnelly MAP, et al. Comparison of home antigen testing with RT-PCR and viral culture during the course of SARS-CoV-2 infection. *JAMA Intern Med*. 2022;182(7):701–709. doi:10.1001/jamainternmed.2022.1827

CHAPTER 3

How do I read an epidemiologic article?

Reading a journal article can feel overwhelming. Many students find that they spend hours reading an article, only to get to the end and realize that they don't really understand it at all. The language can be highly technical, and it is easy to get lost in the details. It is no surprise that students often report reading journal articles as one of the most time-consuming and difficult parts of their coursework and research. More than once, I've had a student tell me that reading a journal article gave them anxiety or made them cry. As we've said, though, being able to critically read and evaluate a scientific journal article is one of the most important skills of an epidemiologist or an evidence-based health practitioner. Fortunately, you can develop your skills and learn to read articles thoroughly and efficiently (and without tears).

Where do I begin?

Journal articles in epidemiology, public health, and medicine typically follow a common structure, in which specific information goes in specific places (Table 3.1). Additionally, collaborative groups have developed guidelines for reporting study results in scientific manuscripts, and many journals now require authors to follow these guidelines when writing their articles. STROBE,[1] for observational studies, and CONSORT,[2] for randomized trials, are two of the most relevant guidelines for epidemiologists (we also will cover PRISMA, for systematic reviews and meta-analyses in Chapter 11). You can read all about STROBE and CONSORT and access checklists and other helpful resources on the EQUATOR (Enhancing the Quality and Transparency of Health Research) Network's website (www.equator-network. org). I have also summarized the key ideas of these reporting guidelines in Box 3.1.

DOI: 10.4324/9781003637899-4

> **Box 3.1**
>
> **Highlights of STROBE and CONSORT publication guidelines**
>
> *STROBE*
>
> STrengthening the Reporting of OBservational studies in Epidemiology
>
>   Specifies unique reporting standards for different study designs, i.e., cross-sectional, case-control, prospective cohort, but generally include:
>
> - Clearly define exposure, outcome, potential confounders, and effect modifiers.
> - Describe data measurements and statistical methods for subgroup analyses, interactions, and missing data.
> - Present the main findings of the study, e.g., study participants, outcome events, summary measures of association.
> - Interpret the study findings in the context of existing evidence.
>
> *CONSORT*
>
> CONsolidated Standards Of Reporting Trials
>
> - Provide a detailed description of the trial design, including recruitment, eligibility criteria, and outcome measurements.
> - Identify the methods and procedures used for randomization.
> - Report the results of the trial, e.g., baseline data, outcomes, and estimations of measures of association.
> - Interpret the trial results, including implications, generalizability, and quality of existing evidence.

Table 3.1 General structure of an epidemiology journal article

Section	Description
Abstract	A brief (~250 words), but complete, summary of the article that is often "structured" with headings such as *Background, Objective, Methods, Results, Conclusion.*
Introduction	Provides the background and rationale for the study. Typically brief (~3–4 paragraphs) yet provides sufficient background for readers to understand the issue, the gap in the current knowledge, why addressing that gap is important, and how the study addresses that gap. The study's purpose is typically stated in the last paragraph.
Methods	Provides specific details on all relevant aspects of a study's methodology. Typically subdivided into sections such as *Study Population, Data Collection, Laboratory Measures,* and *Statistical Analysis.* If a study utilizes a population that has been reported on previously, the article may refer back to prior publications with detailed descriptions of recruitment procedures and other methodological details and provide only a brief overview in the present article.

(Continued)

Table 3.1 (*Continued*)

Section	Description
Results	Reports the study's findings objectively and without interpretation. Provides text to accompany and explain tables and figures. Reported results should match the analyses described in the Methods section.
Discussion	Summarizes the study's findings, typically starting with a brief (2–3 sentences) statement of the key results. Compares the study's results with those previously reported, noting similarities and differences and discussing possible explanations for differences. Provides an assessment of the study's strengths and limitations and how these impact the validity of the results. Interprets the meaning of the results and discusses their public health and/or clinical significance. Suggests directions for future research.
Tables/figures	Summarizes the results of the statistical analysis in tabular or graphical forms. Most journals limit research articles to 4–6 tables/figures. Table 1 typically provides descriptive statistics on demographic characteristics, exposure and/or outcome, and other relevant factors.
References	Lists all journal articles and other sources cited within the article.
Supplementary materials	Sometimes included on the journal's website. May include additional tables and figures with secondary analyses, additional explanation of methods, or deidentified raw data.

Once you understand the structure of epidemiologic articles, reading the article itself becomes much easier. Focusing on reading a section at a time can be helpful to your understanding and can make the process feel a lot less overwhelming. I should also tell you up front that you will need to read some sections of the article multiple times. And, you might need to read the entire article more than once depending on how much you know about the topic before you begin. You don't need to be an expert on a topic to effectively critically analyze a scientific article, but you do need to have a basic understanding of what is already known and what remains to be understood. The Introduction should provide sufficient background for you to understand the purpose and significance of the study (and if it doesn't, you can comment on that in your critical analysis!). On the other hand, if you have a limited (or no) prior knowledge of the topic, you may find that reading (or at least skimming) a review article on the topic first will help you to understand the field and provide important context as you read and critically analyze the article at hand.

Before you sit down to read the full article, you should first read its Abstract. Nearly all articles will include an Abstract, which is typically a 250-word summary of the key points. Reading the Abstract will give you a good overview of the study, including its design, a basic description of the population, the main exposure and outcome, the most important results, and what those findings might mean for the broader field or population. Once you have read the Abstract, you will find that you have a reasonable sense of what the article is going to tell you. This serves as a good scaffold as you read the article itself. Imagine you are reading an article exploring whether depression is a risk factor for breast cancer. After reading the article's Title and Abstract, you know that depression is the primary exposure being studied and breast cancer is the primary outcome under investigation. Now when you read the Methods section, you can think carefully about how both depression (exposure) and breast cancer (outcome) were defined and measured, paying close attention to the relevant strengths and limitations (more to come on how to identify particular strengths and limitations in Chapters 6 and 7).

You should recognize, though, that the Abstract will not tell you everything you need to know about the article. Imagine summarizing your entire thesis into just 250 words—you would definitely have to leave out some really important details! Reading the Abstract is not a substitute for reading the article. The Abstract (usually) will not include any discussion of the strengths and limitations of the study. You will need to carefully read the full article to consider these strengths and limitations (remember, even the best study will have them) and make an accurate conclusion.

Once you have read the Abstract and have a good idea about what to expect, it is time to start reading the actual article. It can be helpful to start a mental list, based on having read the Abstract, of what you want to learn more about. Having these questions in mind can make it easier to go out and find that information. You might think that you need to start from the beginning and read the article all the way through from start to finish. However, sometimes starting in the middle (i.e., Methods) or even the end (i.e., Discussion) can be a lot more helpful to your understanding. Remember, this is not a novel—you won't spoil any of the plot if you skip over the Introduction or read the last paragraph of the Discussion section first.

What you read first after the Abstract might depend on what you already know about the topic and what your goals are when reading the article. If this is a completely new area for you, then reading the Introduction will give you a good sense of what is currently known about the topic and why the research question at hand is important. For example, an article about an Ebola outbreak began by describing the number of cases and deaths that occurred in the region and why researching pathways of disease transmission is important for preventing future outbreaks.[3]

If you already have a solid background in the topic area, then you might be able to skim the Introduction or even skip to its final paragraph, which typically includes a statement of the study's purpose and primary research question. At a minimum, you'll want to identify how the authors define their research question and purpose. Knowing this information will help you consider how well the study addresses the stated question.

Why do I need to read the Methods section so carefully?

Personally, I feel that the Methods section is the most important section for you to read and focus on when critically evaluating an epidemiologic article. This is because the Methods section is where you learn about all the factors that affect the internal and external validity of the study (see Chapter 2 for definition and discussion of these terms): what study design is used? Who is in the study population? How is the exposure measured? How is the outcome measured? How are the data analyzed? If you can focus your effort on carefully reading and understanding the Methods section, then understanding the Results and Discussion sections will be far easier.

What do you need to think about as you read the Methods section? Chapters 4–8 will take you through all the detailed questions and considerations, but here I present the big picture. As you read the Methods section, you will want to understand the key details about each part of the study. You will want to take notes as you go—write down the key facts and your thoughts about any potential for bias or error that you notice (in other words, take notes on any limitations you identify). Just as importantly, write down any strengths of the methodology that serve to prevent or reduce the potential for bias, confounding, or error.

Again: there is no such thing as a perfect study! Every study will have some potential for bias, confounding, or error. In fact, most studies will have more than one issue. Typically, though, only a few of these issues will have a meaningful impact on the study's validity. Just because you recognize that there is a bias present doesn't mean it has a major impact on the study's findings. Sometimes there is a small likelihood that the issue meaningfully affected the results.

Take as an example a study exploring purported associations between vaccination against severe acute respiratory syndrome coronavirus 2 (SARS-CoV-2, the virus that caused the COVID-19 pandemic) and fertility.[4] The investigators asked participants to self-report whether they had ever been infected with SARS-CoV-2 and also whether they had ever received a COVID-19 vaccine. As we will see in future chapters, self-reporting almost always comes with a potential for measurement error. It is possible that some participants reported being vaccinated when they actually were not vaccinated, or that they had never had COVID-19, when they actually had been infected with the SARS-CoV-2 virus. However, because participants reported on their COVID-19 illness and vaccination status *before* they were pregnant, it is very unlikely that any inaccuracies in reporting would be related to whether or not they were able to conceive (in epidemiology jargon, differential misclassification of exposure is unlikely), and therefore, as the authors point out in their Discussion section, the estimated risk ratios are unbiased.[4]

As you read an article and identify its limitations, your job is to figure out which limitations are the most likely to have impacted the results, and potentially by how much. I find it helpful to think about putting issues into three buckets: minor, moderate, and major (Figure 3.1). We will talk more about these buckets and how to distinguish between minor, moderate, and major issues as we work through Chapters 4–8.

For now, as you read the Methods section, think about how different issues might have arisen and how they might have impacted the results. Would the bias/confounding/ error tend to make it more likely that an association was found (in epidemiology jargon, we would call this "bias away from the null hypothesis") or would it make it less likely to find an association ("bias toward the null hypothesis")? How big of an effect might the error have had (in epidemiology jargon, we would refer to this as its impact on the *magnitude* of the association)? Going back to our example of COVID-19 infection and vaccination in relation to couples' ability to conceive,[4] the potential error caused by inaccurate self-reports of infection and vaccination status would be similar between those who did and did not become pregnant (because the reports were made before anyone was pregnant, and because there is no reason to believe that one's ability to accurately report would be related to their future ability to conceive). This type of error, which we described as **non-differential misclassification of exposure** in Chapter 2,

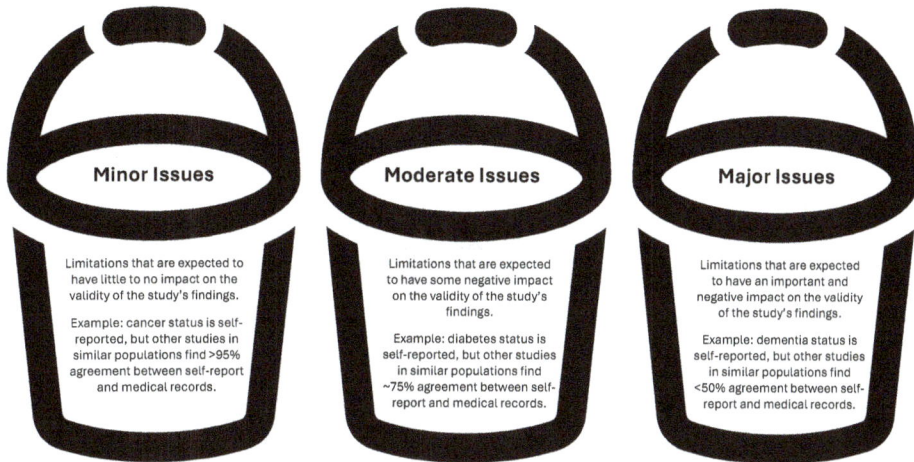

Figure 3.1 Conceptualizing the limitations of a study as fitting into buckets describing their impact on study results can be helpful in evaluating threats to validity.

tends to bias results toward the null hypothesis. Furthermore, because COVID-19 testing, including self-testing, was widely available by the time the study began and because people tend to be highly accurate in reporting vaccination status (the authors note that prior studies of influenza vaccination showed 97% agreement between self-reports and medical records), we can conclude that any reporting error would be small and unlikely to have a substantial impact on the study's findings. In other words, it is still important to make note of this limitation, but we likely would put it into our "minor issues" bucket.

How can I thoroughly evaluate the article for all the possible threats to validity?

You might think that this process would be easiest if you had a list of every single bias and then just checked off "yes" or "no" for each one. I'd caution against this approach, though. As of this writing, *The Catalogue of Bias* (https://catalogofbias.org/) identifies more than sixty different types of biases that can affect health studies. And, since most of these will not be present in any given study, going through each one would be a lot of wasted effort. We are far better off focusing on the issues that are most likely to be present and are likely to substantially impact the results.

As you write your critical analysis, you don't need to discuss in detail the issues that are unlikely to be present or those issues that only minimally influence the estimated associations. For example, survival bias (where both the exposure and outcome being studied affect individuals' probability of surviving and thus being alive and able to be included in the study) is unlikely to significantly impact a prospective study of physical activity and behavioral issues among a population of healthy children. On the other hand, a retrospective study exploring associations between alcohol use and motor vehicle crashes could be strongly affected by survival bias, since people who are heavy alcohol drinkers might be more likely to die in a car accident and therefore wouldn't be available for you to study. In upcoming chapters, we will think through each of the main components of the study's methodology and learn to critically analyze these methods and focus on identifying threats to validity.

A systematic approach for reading and taking notes on an article

First, let's come up with a plan for reading the article and taking notes in a way that supports your critical thinking and, ultimately, the writing of your critical analysis. Using a systematic approach and a standard set of questions will help guide your reading, focus your attention on the most relevant details, and ensure that you don't miss anything.

We will use my System for Taking notes on ARticles (the STAR template; see Appendix A, and also available as a fillable template in the online supplementary material) as our companion as we read journal articles. As we work through Chapters 4–8, we will complete the template for the Mirick et al.[5] article that we introduced in Chapter 1. For now, let's examine the overall structure of the STAR template.

You'll see that the first piece of information to record is a complete citation for the article. This is extremely important, as you will need this information when you write your critical analysis and any time you reference the study in your writing and presentations (think: grant applications, research papers, presentations). At the same time, I highly recommend that you add the reference to whatever citation management software you prefer to use (many academics prefer Zotero or Mendeley, which are typically available for free through your institution's library).

The STAR template is organized as a series of tables. There are separate tables for each of the key methodological components of the study: study purpose and design (Section 1), study population (Section 2), exposure assessment (Section 3), outcome assessment (Section 4), statistical analysis (Section 5), results and conclusions (Section 6), and a final table for your own overall assessment (Section 7). Sections 1–6 are set up the same way: in the left-hand column, you will record details about the study, and in the right-hand column, you will add your analysis. The questions in the left-hand column are designed to make sure you understand and take notes on the key methodological details. Here, you are to record just the facts; keep your own ideas and interpretations out of this column.

I recommend being careful in noting whether you are paraphrasing what the authors wrote or if you are including a direct quotation. It can be very challenging to effectively paraphrase details of study methodology, and many students find that they write down verbatim how the authors described these details. This is fine, but make sure that you indicate this in your notes so that you don't forget to paraphrase these details when you write your critical analysis later. I find that it is most helpful to include some direct quotations, identified using quotation marks, in my notes. This way, I am certain that I have recorded the methods accurately, and I also know that I need to paraphrase when I write my critical analysis. I have seen many students unintentionally plagiarize when they write their papers, often due to sloppy note-taking.

Once you have recorded the details using the questions in the left-hand column, answer the questions in the right-hand column to develop your critical analysis. The right-hand column is designed to help you think through the strengths and limitations of the methods and results, using a series of questions that are appropriate for each major aspect of the study design. Note, though, that a single template cannot possibly cover every important aspect of every published study. The questions included are meant as guides to help you think about each component, but the template also includes space to add additional strengths and/or limitations that you feel are relevant and merit inclusion in your critical analysis.

After you have completed Sections 1–6, Section 7 will help you develop an overall assessment of the article. Here, you will record any potential conflicts of interest that you have noted. The primary focus of this section, though, is to think through the strengths and limitations that you identified in Sections 1–6, and to highlight the most important ones. Yes, this will feel quite repetitive since you have already noted these strengths and limitations in Sections 1–6. But, recording them in a single spot will be incredibly helpful as you sit down to write your critical analysis paper. Section 7 is designed to make you step back and see the forest through the trees to evaluate the overall quality of the article. Here, I give you three options for rating the article: poor, good, and excellent. We each have our own internal rating system and understanding of what separates a "poor" article from a "good" article, and it is not my goal to change that. Two (or more) people who are well-trained can evaluate the same article and come to different assessments about its relative strengths and limitations and their impact on internal validity. This is part of science! The STAR template asks you to record *your* characterization of the article's overall quality, and you should use your own internal definitions of what is "poor," "good," or "excellent." We'll cover how to evaluate article quality in Chapter 9. These assessments are meant to be helpful to you as you weigh the article's findings in your future writing and presentations. Note, though, that if you do write a systematic review and/or meta-analysis, you'll want to define your rating system so that you can apply it consistently across the articles you read. More to come on systematic reviews in Chapter 11.

Finally, Section 7 asks you to write a very brief summary of the article's key features and conclusions, based on your assessment of its strengths and limitations. This is not easy to do within five sentences. Most of the time, though, you will not be writing about the article and its findings in a full-length critical analysis without page restrictions. More commonly, you will be referring to the article's findings in the Introduction and Discussion sections of your own research articles or in the Significance section of a grant application. In either case, you will need to write a succinct summary of the article's key findings and its validity. Scientific writing tends to be very concise, and it takes time and practice to develop this skill. Including a brief paragraph summarizing your critical analysis of the article right on your note-taking template will be very helpful to you in the future.

STAR in action: examining the study purpose and design in Mirick et al.

In Chapters 4–8, we will include a completed example of the STAR template, based on the Mirick et al.[5] article. Here, we start by completing Section 1 for Mirick et al. (Table 3.2).

The article by Mirick et al.[5] sought to evaluate the association between antiperspirant and deodorant use and breast cancer risk, using a population-based case-control study design. The authors conducted this study in response to persistent rumors of a link between antiperspirants and breast cancer risk, despite a lack of rigorous scientific evidence. The researchers leveraged data from an existing case-control study, which

Table 3.2 Completed STAR template Section 1: "Study Purpose and Design" for Mirick et al. (2002)[5]

1. Study purpose and design	
Describe (i.e., report just the facts described in the article)	*Critique (i.e., think through strengths/limitations of the methods and results, address the key questions listed, and add additional comments as needed)*
What is the objective/ purpose of the study? **To evaluate the association between antiperspirant/ deodorant use and breast cancer risk in females**	Is sufficient justification for the stated objective/purpose provided? Is there a plausible biologic or theoretical mechanism provided? **Yes, as stated in the article, there have been many media/ internet reports that claim an association between underarm hygiene and breast cancer. Authors note that rumors persist despite lack of rigorous evidence.**
What type of study design was used? **Population-based case-control study**	Is this an appropriate design for addressing the stated objective/purpose? Why or why not? **Case-controlv study is an appropriate choice because:** ■ **Useful with rare outcomes (like breast cancer).** ■ **Can evaluate multiple exposures.** ■ **Can be conducted more quickly than a prospective cohort.** ■ **Useful for diseases with long latency period (like breast cancer).** **Potential concerns though:** ■ **Lack of temporality** ■ **Prone to bias (e.g., selection bias, recall bias—see below)** Note any additional comments: ■ None noted

allowed them to evaluate an additional exposure in relation to breast cancer risk and perform the study efficiently. However, this design raises concerns regarding lack of temporality as well as a strong potential for selection bias and recall bias. We will evaluate the extent to which such biases affected the results as we continue our critical analysis.

Activities

Find a recently published observational study or randomized controlled trial on a topic of interest to you. You might consider identifying an article from one of the journals that you explored in the Activities from Chapter 1.

1. Create an outline of the article by identifying the purpose and/or main topic of each paragraph (i.e., don't write *what* the authors said—write *why* the authors said it).
2. Read the article and complete the left-hand side of Sections 1–6 of the STAR template to help you abstract the key information from the article.

3. Using one of the reporting guidelines discussed in this chapter (e.g., STROBE for observational studies, CONSORT for randomized controlled trials), evaluate the article. How well does the reporting of the study adhere to the guidelines?

References

1. STROBE. STROBE. Accessed November 17, 2023. https://www.strobe-statement.org/
2. Schulz KF, Altman DG, Moher D, CONSORT Group. CONSORT 2010 statement: Updated guidelines for reporting parallel group randomized trials. *Ann Intern Med*. 2010; 152(11):726–732. doi:10.7326/0003–4819-152-11–201006010-00232
3. Robert A, Edmunds WJ, Watson CH, et al. Determinants of transmission risk during the late stage of the West African Ebola epidemic. *Am J Epidemiol*. 2019;188(7):1319–1327. doi:10.1093/aje/kwz090
4. Wesselink AK, Hatch EE, Rothman KJ, et al. A prospective cohort study of COVID-19 vaccination, SARS-CoV-2 infection, and fertility. *Am J Epidemiol*. 2022;191(8):1383–1395. doi:10.1093/aje/kwac011
5. Mirick DK, Davis S, Thomas DB. Antiperspirant use and the risk of breast cancer. *J Natl Cancer Inst*. 2002;94(20):1578–1580. doi:10.1093/jnci/94.20.1578

What study design was used?

One of the first elements you will need to identify in the research article is the study design that was used. This is a key methodological feature. It is so key, in fact, that most introductory epidemiology courses are organized around teaching students the fundamental study designs. We will cover them here as well, but I will assume that you already know the "nuts and bolts" of each one and can identify the study design that was used when you read the description of the study methodology.

Here, we will focus on how the study design that is chosen impacts the potential internal validity. Not all study designs are created equal. Different study designs are more (or less) susceptible to certain types of bias and error. We will need to be on the lookout for these issues as we engage in a critical analysis of the study. When you read a case-control study, for example, it is helpful to think about the most common potential issues and then read closely to see how (or if) these potential limitations are addressed within the study.

Generally speaking, we can put epidemiologic study designs into two categories: descriptive studies and analytic studies. Descriptive studies have the primary purpose of *describing* what is going on in a population (or an individual) with respect to distributions of exposures and health outcomes (e.g., diseases, screening behaviors, and mortality). These studies can be thought of as hypothesis generating. Analytic studies have the primary purpose of *analyzing* associations between exposures and health outcomes. These studies can be thought of as hypothesis testing.

There is an accepted hierarchy of strength of study designs in relation to causality (Figure 4.1). Just because an article you are reading uses a design lower on the hierarchy, though, doesn't mean that you should dismiss its findings out of hand. It is important to note that this hierarchy assumes the study has been perfectly executed such that the internal validity is as high as possible given its design. In practice, this is not always the case. A rigorously designed case-control study could certainly have higher internal validity and provide more information about causality than a poorly designed prospective cohort study with major limitations affecting its internal validity.

DOI: 10.4324/9781003637899-5

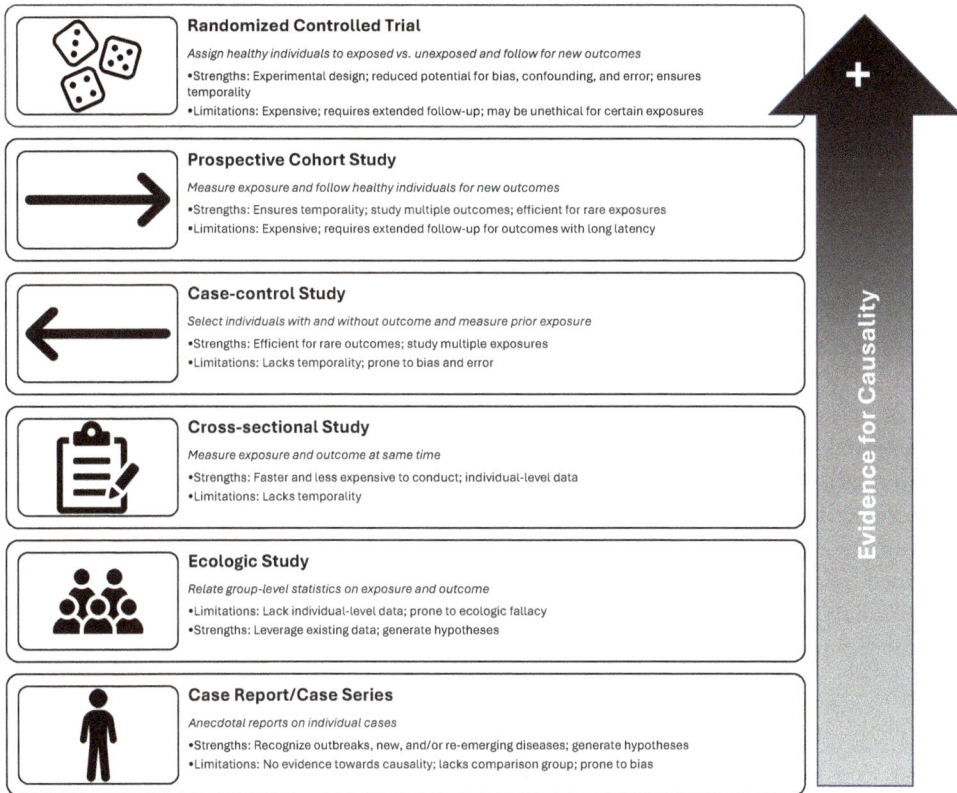

Figure 4.1 Hierarchy of epidemiologic study designs.

Also, it is important to recognize that not all research questions can be answered with all study designs. For example, a prospective cohort study lasting 60 years is not always feasible, and a randomized controlled trial (RCT) evaluating smoking as the exposure would not be ethical. As we consider the strengths and limitations of the various study designs, we also will explore how and why researchers select one design over another when conducting a study.

What are the descriptive study designs?

Case report/series

A **case report** is just as its name would suggest: the detailed report of a single case. Often, more than one similar case is written up, with this study design referred to as a **case series**. Such studies are very common and are highly important in medical literature. Some leading medical journals (e.g., *New England Journal of Medicine*) even devote a section of each issue to case reports/series. It is far less common to see this study design within an epidemiology journal.

These studies cannot tell us anything conclusive about exposure–disease relationships within the population—they only study a small number of individuals and lack a comparison group—but by providing detailed descriptions of unusual cases of diseases, these designs can help to identify new diseases and their causes. While you should never rely on a case report or case series for demonstrating causality, you should not write them off as entirely useless either. In fact, case reports/series were critical in recognizing important epidemics, including HIV/AIDS[1] and West Nile,[2] and they play important roles in identifying outbreaks of foodborne illness (e.g., a case series recognized an *Escherichia coli* outbreak that was later linked to flour[3]). These initial, anecdotal reports can suggest populations at the highest risk as well as potential risk factors to be explored in subsequent analytic studies.

Surveillance

Likewise, disease **surveillance** studies cannot test hypotheses nor demonstrate causality, yet surveillance is critical for identifying outbreaks, epidemics, and changing patterns of disease. In the U.S., the Centers for Disease Control and Prevention oversees the National Notifiable Diseases Surveillance System (NNDSS), a passive surveillance system that tracks diseases where case reporting is mandatory.[4] The NNDSS is critical for recognizing important public health threats, including foodborne illnesses and lead poisoning. Continual surveillance of key diseases and conditions ensures that they are identified quickly and early. This reporting brings them to the attention of public health professionals, who can then investigate to identify causes and intervene to reduce further morbidity and mortality.

Ecologic study

Studies that examine correlations between distributions of exposures and outcomes across populations are referred to as **ecologic studies.** You have probably seen examples of ecologic studies and not even realized it; these studies are often presented as plots, showing how the prevalence of a risk factor in a group relates to the prevalence or incidence of an outcome within that same group. Very often the unit of observation is defined geographically, such as by state or country, though other definitions for groups can be used. Ecologic studies can often be conducted quickly and at low cost, as they generally take advantage of previously collected data. Publicly available data on populations from the World Health Organization, the U.S. Census Bureau, or other governmental agencies are often used to conduct ecologic studies. For example, an ecologic study demonstrated a positive association between air pollution and lung cancer incidence and mortality across 100 counties of the U.S. state of North Carolina.[5]

The key defining characteristic of an ecologic study is that the unit of observation is a group, not an individual. Because data are not available on individuals, ecologic studies are highly prone to **ecologic fallacy.** An ecologic fallacy is when associations observed at the group level do not hold true when similar associations are evaluated using individual-level data. Essentially, we have no idea if those who are exposed are also those with the outcome (or, if those who are not exposed are also those without the outcome), because we only have data on the groups as a whole, not on the individuals who make up the groups. For example, ecologic studies showed a strong positive trend between dietary fat intake and breast cancer mortality[6]; however, rigorously conducted and internally valid analytic studies have failed to demonstrate a statistically significant, causal relationship between dietary fat and breast cancer risk, even in a meta-analysis of prospective cohort studies evaluating this association.[7]

We saw another example of an ecologic study in the McGrath[8] article on antiperspirants and breast cancer, when the author used a positive correlation between U.S. sales of antiperspirants/deodorants from 1940 to 2000 and U.S. breast cancer rates over the same time period as support for the hypothesis that these products may be contributing to breast cancer incidence. The problem (one among many) is that we have no way of knowing whether the *individuals* using antiperspirants/deodorants were also the ones being diagnosed with breast cancer. And, we have no way of adjusting for the many potential factors (e.g., age, race, menstrual/reproductive history) that likely confound any relationship between antiperspirant/deodorant use and breast cancer risk. The saying "correlation does not equal causation" may be a cliché, but it is indeed true. While ecologic studies can be helpful for generating hypotheses, we must always be careful not to overinterpret their findings as evidence for (or against) causality.

Cross-sectional study

Cross-sectional studies can be thought of as a snapshot of a population's health at a given time. For this reason, some epidemiologists refer to cross-sectional studies as "prevalence studies." Cross-sectional studies can be relatively fast, inexpensive, and straightforward to conduct. Researchers can measure exposure status and outcome status on a defined study population, gather individual-level data, and then estimate associations between exposure prevalence and outcome prevalence within that population.

When I am teaching, I often conduct a cross-sectional study on the spot by asking students to respond to a questionnaire asking them if they own a pet (yes/no) and if they have asthma (yes/no). It can really be that simple. If I wanted, I could also ask them questions about potential confounders and then adjust for those in our analysis. One problem with this approach that we just cannot get around is temporality. Because I am measuring the prevalence of pet ownership (exposure) and asthma (outcome) at the same time, I have no way of knowing which came first: pet ownership or asthma. In fact, it is very likely that someone with an asthma diagnosis might subsequently decide not to get a pet after their health care provider tells them that pet dander can exacerbate asthma symptoms.

As with the other descriptive designs we have covered, cross-sectional studies provide limited value for establishing causality. Cross-sectional studies, however, are very useful for estimating the prevalence of exposures and outcomes and for generating causal hypotheses that can then be tested using an analytic study design.

What are the analytic study designs?

Case-control study

The **case-control study** design is aptly named, as it begins by selecting a group of cases and a separate group of controls. Then, exposure is measured in both the cases and in the controls. While its name is straightforward, conducting these studies can be quite challenging. The case-control design, as your introductory epidemiology professor will tell you, is excellent when you have a rare disease and/or a disease with a long latency period. For example, if the lifetime risk of ovarian cancer is only 1 in 87 females and takes 10–20 years to develop to a point where it can be clinically diagnosed,[9] you could spend your entire career (and a lot of money) enrolling participants into a prospective cohort study and following them until enough cases are diagnosed for you to study. It is far more efficient (both in time and money) to instead start by identifying cases that are newly diagnosed and at the same time enroll a comparable group of "healthy" people without the disease of interest. Then, the exposure status is determined for both cases and controls. Seems quite simple, right?

The case-control design can be incredibly powerful (e.g., it was critical for establishing smoking as a cause of lung cancer[10]), but this design also is highly prone to bias and error. Researchers must carefully design case-control studies using methodology that minimizes the opportunity for bias and error as much as possible.

Here, let's focus on three of the most important aspects of conducting a case-control study: (1) selecting cases, (2) selecting controls, and (3) assessing exposure status. These are places where there is a high potential for bias and error to creep in, and so it will be very important to pay attention to the details of these aspects as you read articles that use a case-control study design.

Selecting cases

As you know from your introductory epidemiology course, it is important that case-control studies use a standard case definition and enroll newly diagnosed (i.e., "incident") cases. What you may not remember is *why* this is so important.

Using a standard case definition promotes the validity of our outcome assessment—we know that a participant enrolled as a case truly has the outcome of interest. This is especially important in multicenter studies: we need to be certain that a case enrolled from one clinical site meets the same case criteria as a case enrolled from another clinical site. The standard case definition can reduce outcome misclassification, which we will talk about in depth in Chapter 7.

Enrolling incident cases helps to promote internal validity by reducing survival bias (a form of selection bias). Survival bias occurs when the exposure influences disease survival. As a result, the exposure distribution among those who *survive* the disease ends up being quite different than the exposure distribution among those who *die from* the disease. For this reason, it is important to enroll cases into the study as soon after diagnosis as possible; this is especially critical for diseases with a short survival (e.g., pancreatic cancer, which has a 1-year survival rate of only 32%[11]). If the study excludes deceased cases, then a survival bias can result, and the estimated association between exposure and disease incidence would be biased. There are important logistical issues too—including prevalent cases, which make it challenging to measure the exposure during a relevant window of time; prevalent cases are farther out from diagnosis and, therefore, farther from the period of time when exposure could impact the development of the disease or condition.

Other forms of selection bias can occur within case-control studies as well. Recall that selection bias occurs when the probability of enrollment into the study is somehow related to exposure and outcome status. Imagine we recruit cases of asthma from patients admitted to a hospital for an asthma attack. We know that not all cases of asthma require hospitalization, even among those cases that seek care at the emergency department. Therefore, the hospitalized cases are likely to be the most severe cases. If the exposure of interest is associated with the *severity* of the disease, then the probability of exposure would be linked to the probability of hospitalization, and, therefore, the probability of selection into the study. In other words, we have a problem. We might wrongly conclude that an exposure is related to overall asthma risk, when what we are really studying is "risk of asthma attack severe enough to result in hospitalization."

Selecting controls

Identifying and enrolling a comparable control group is one of the most challenging parts of a case-control study. It is critical that controls are selected from the same source population that produced the cases and that they meet the same eligibility criteria as the cases (except for having the outcome of interest, of course). A helpful approach to evaluating if controls are comparable to cases is the "would" test: if a member of the control group were diagnosed with the disease under study, *would* they have been eligible to be selected as a case? If the answer is no, then the control group is not comparable to the cases.

Additionally, we need to be certain that controls are free of the disease being studied. This often requires screening them for the disease in some way. Screening could be as simple as asking them (e.g., do you have asthma?). In some cases, though, screening may require reviewing medical records or administering a screening test (e.g., females with a normal screening mammogram often form the control group for case-control studies of breast cancer). Because many diseases may be asymptomatic in early stages, it is important to know the natural history of the disease under study. This will facilitate appropriate methods for verifying that controls are free of disease. If controls with undetected disease are enrolled, this outcome misclassification will reduce the internal validity of the study (more on why in Chapter 7).

We also need to ensure that controls are at-risk for the disease being studied. This is key to ensuring that they are truly a fair comparison group for the cases and that the prevalence of exposure in the control group reflects its distribution in the target population. For some conditions, it will be obvious that certain groups need to be excluded because they are not at-risk (e.g., biologic females should not be included in a case-control study of prostate cancer). Oftentimes, individuals' at-risk status may be less clear and require additional screening. For example, females who have had their uterus removed (i.e., hysterectomy) would not be at risk for endometrial cancer. Therefore, a study seeking to evaluate risk factors for endometrial cancer would need to screen potential participants for whether or not they have an intact uterus, either by asking them to self-report or reviewing medical records for prior hysterectomy.

Many case-control studies use matching to ensure comparability, reduce confounding, and increase statistical efficiency. In an individually matched case-control study, for every case that is selected, a control (or a set of controls) is selected that has the same values for the matching criteria. Common matching criteria include age, race, ethnicity, and biological sex. Because the selection of controls is dependent upon the selection of the cases, the observations are no longer independent of one another. As a result, special statistical methods that account for this dependence are needed (e.g., paired t-tests, conditional logistic regression). Frequency matched case-control studies seek to enroll case and control groups that have the same distributions of matching criteria overall, but individual cases and controls are not specifically matched to one another. This approach has the advantage of ensuring comparability while still maintaining independence of the observations and allowing for traditional statistical approaches to be used (e.g., unpaired t-tests, unconditional logistic regression). Also, matching factors in a frequency-matched study can still be studied for their association with the outcome (or other outcomes in future analyses), whereas this is not possible if cases and controls are individually matched on a given factor. If, for example, cases and controls are matched on biological sex, then biological sex cannot be explored as a risk factor for the disease, since the cases and their matched control(s) have the same biological sex.

Assessing exposure status

Because case-control studies are retrospective, exposure assessment can be incredibly challenging and highly prone to bias and error. Specifically, case-control studies are very susceptible to recall bias, because cases and controls may have a different recollection of their exposure histories. Many case-control studies ask participants to self-report their previous exposure history. Depending on the timeframe involved, this may be more or less accurate. Imagine being asked to report on your intake of fruits and vegetables during childhood; young adults might be able to report this reasonably well, but older adults might have a lot of trouble remembering what they ate ≥40 years ago. While any errors in exposure assessment can negatively impact internal validity, these errors are especially problematic when the accuracy of exposure assessment is different between cases and controls (in epidemiology jargon, this is called differential misclassification of exposure). Exposure misclassification ends up being a big potential issue in case-control studies; more to come on this topic in Chapter 6.

Prospective cohort study

The design of **prospective cohort studies** is straightforward: a group of participants without the outcome of interest (but who are at-risk for the outcome) are enrolled, their exposure status is assessed to determine if they are exposed or unexposed, and then they are followed forward in time to determine who develops the outcome and who does not. Prospective cohort studies are generally regarded as the observational study design with the greatest potential to offer evidence toward causality. It is easy to understand why: prospective cohort studies have the appropriate temporality. We know the exposure occurred before the outcome, because none of the participants had the outcome when the study began. This is a key feature for establishing causality that the designs reviewed previously have all lacked. Additionally, prospective cohort studies can be designed to evaluate multiple exposures and multiple outcomes, adding to their usefulness. Also, issues of differential misclassification of the exposure (when the accuracy of exposure assessment differs by outcome status) are less likely in a prospective cohort study, because the exposure is assessed before the outcomes develop.

There are important challenges to conducting a prospective cohort study, however. For one thing, these studies often require large numbers of participants, even for diseases that we may think of as common. Let's use breast cancer as an example, which is the most commonly diagnosed invasive cancer among U.S. females (and a frequent topic of discussion within the lay press and on social media), yet it is still a "rare" disease. Imagine that you want to conduct a prospective cohort study to evaluate risk factors for breast cancer. Your biostatistician colleague has calculated that you will need 500 new breast cancer diagnoses within your cohort to have sufficient statistical power to test your hypotheses (more to come on statistical power in Chapter 8). If you could only run your study for, say, 1 year, then you might decide to enroll women at the age when their risk of breast cancer diagnosis is highest. For women ages ≥65, the breast cancer incidence rate is 439 cases diagnosed per 100,000 women each year. Some more quick math tells us that in order to generate 500 incident breast cancer cases, we would need to enroll $(439/100,000)^{-1} \times 500 = 113,895$ participants age ≥65 and follow them for 1 year. A massive undertaking indeed. Hopefully, you get the point: prospective cohort studies require huge amounts of resources, especially financial resources.

The internal validity of a prospective cohort study will be affected by our usual suspects: who is included in the study population, how accurately the exposure is measured, and how accurately the outcome is measured. A key threat to internal validity in prospective cohort studies is that selection bias can occur if loss to follow-up differs based on the participant's exposure and outcome status. Imagine a study where 90% of participants with the exposure who *do not* develop disease are followed for the full study period, yet only 75% of exposed participants who *do* develop the disease are followed for the full study period (the rest drop out of the study before we know their diagnosis status). This difference in follow-up rates would mean that our study population includes an artificially greater proportion of exposed individuals who do not develop the outcome. More to come on selection bias in Chapter 5. For now, suffice it to say that we need to pay careful attention to the follow-up rates when we read a prospective cohort study.

Retrospective cohort study

You may be wondering about **retrospective cohort studies**. Students often find the term "retrospective cohort" to be confusing. In a retrospective (or "historical") cohort study, both exposure and outcome have occurred *before* the investigators began the study. Typically, these studies rely on records (e.g., military, school, occupational, and medical) to assess both exposure and outcome status. It is important to recognize that in a retrospective cohort study, the exposure and outcome were assessed in real time; therefore, they are not susceptible to recall bias. The "retrospective" piece refers to the records themselves—all the data were collected before the investigation began. Occupational studies are often conducted using a retrospective cohort design. For example, a retrospective cohort study reported that occupational exposure to inorganic dust and fumes slightly increased the risk of chronic kidney disease among construction workers.[12] The increased availability of electronic health records in recent decades is leading to a resurgence of retrospective cohort studies.

Retrospective cohort studies are ideal for rare exposures where detailed records on exposure and outcomes are available on a defined study population. The reliance on the availability of prior records, however, also can present challenges. Usually, these records were not collected with an epidemiologic study in mind, and the data can be messy to work with, to say the least.

Also, it is important to note that using previously collected data from a prospective cohort study to answer a new question *is not* a retrospective cohort study. Such a study would more accurately be described as a secondary analysis of a prospective cohort study. It is still a prospective cohort study because the original investigators enrolled a study population without the outcome, assessed their exposure status, and then followed them forward in time. This is different from a retrospective cohort study, where all the data on exposure and outcome were collected before the investigators began the study.

Variations on a theme: additional observational study designs

The case-control and prospective cohort designs have been used as building blocks to create additional study designs: nested case-control and case-cohort studies. Ideally, these variations take the strengths of both designs and minimize their limitations, gaining efficiency in the process.

In a **nested case-control study**, researchers begin with a defined study population enrolled in a prospective cohort study. For every case of the outcome that is diagnosed within the cohort during the follow-up period, one (or more) control is selected from among the study population. Controls are required to have been alive and at risk for the outcome at the time of the case's diagnosis, and they are typically matched on important confounding factors, such as age, sex, and/or race/ethnicity. Don't let the words "case-control" in the name fool you: this design avoids many of the issues associated with selection of cases and controls and with retrospectively assessing exposure that we discussed earlier. Its strengths and limitations are much closer to a prospective cohort study.

A **case-cohort study** is somewhat similar. Researchers select cases diagnosed with the outcome of interest within a prospective cohort. Instead of matching controls to each case, however, a "sub-cohort" is created from a randomly selected group of participants available at the study baseline. An advantage of this design is that this same sub-cohort can be used for future research studies with different outcomes, because the sub-cohort selection was done completely independently of the case group.

Nested case-control and case-cohort designs are often used when laboratory analysis of biological samples is required for exposure assessment. Both designs can substantially reduce the costs associated with running laboratory assays on a full cohort. Imagine your team is interested in studying a biomarker that costs $150 per sample to measure. Measuring that biomarker on an entire cohort of 25,000 participants would cost $3,750,000! However, if you selected the 500 cases of your outcome that were diagnosed within that cohort, and then another 500 matched controls (or a sub-cohort of 500 participants), your costs to measure the biomarker in 1000 samples would be $150,000—far more feasible than the original price tag. For example, a nested case-control study evaluated whether endocrine-disrupting chemicals were associated with postmenopausal breast cancer risk within the prospective Women's Health Initiative cohort,[13] and a case-cohort study within the American Cancer Society's Cancer Prevention Study II cohort explored associations between perfluoroalkyl substances and prostate cancer[14] as well as kidney and bladder cancers.[15]

Randomized controlled trials

RCTs have long been considered the gold standard of epidemiologic study designs. They are the closest epidemiologists come to designing experiments that are as well-controlled as we might achieve in a laboratory. Whereas the previous designs we've reviewed are "observational," meaning that participants decide their exposures for themselves (or, at least, researchers don't decide for them), RCTs are an "experimental" design, where the investigators assign participants to be exposed or not. Readers in medical and other health professional fields will encounter this study design frequently. RCTs are important for establishing evidence-based recommendations for a wide range of topics, from the optimal timing of cancer screening to the efficacy of new treatments.

RCT's reputation as the optimal epidemiologic study design is well-deserved. Randomization of participants to treatment and control groups avoids selection bias and practically eliminates confounding by both measured and unmeasured factors. Because investigators assign the exposure status, they have clear information on the exact nature of the exposure, including timing, dose, and duration. Often participants are unaware of whether they are in the intervention or control group (sometimes referred to as "blinding" or "masking"), making it practically impossible for their reporting of symptoms, etc. to be influenced by knowledge of their exposure. Participants are followed closely and routinely monitored for the development of the outcome(s) of interest. In short, RCTs overcome many of the important limitations to which observational designs are susceptible.

You might be wondering: if RCTs are truly such a strong design, then why would we bother with observational studies at all? It's true that RCTs have numerous strengths, but even RCTs can have limitations. For example, some diseases have extended latency periods, making an RCT very challenging to conduct. In fact, RCTs suffer from similar logistical issues as prospective cohort studies (i.e., substantial resources of time, money, and personnel are needed). An additional limitation is that an RCT isn't always ethical to conduct. For example, you could never conduct an RCT to evaluate whether alcohol use is safe during pregnancy. Even though the observational data are not totally conclusive,[16] there are enough data suggesting that even a low amount of alcohol consumption during pregnancy is harmful to the developing fetus that it would be unethical to randomize someone to consume alcohol while they are pregnant. In cases like these, observational studies are truly the best option for epidemiological studies.

When RCTs are conducted, there are some key issues to look out for when reading journal articles reporting their results. First, adherence to the study treatment protocol can be variable. If results show that the treatment was not effective in preventing the disease, but also that 50% of the comparison group stopped taking the assigned placebo and decided on their own to take the treatment being tested, then we have a big problem with exposure misclassification to address. RCTs are analyzed according to **intention-to-treat analysis,** where we keep participants in their assigned exposure groups even if we know they were non-adherent. As we will learn in Chapter 8, randomization is important for controlling confounding by ensuring that participants in the treatment and comparison groups are similar to one another on other factors that could be related to the exposure and outcome (e.g., age, smoking status). Intention-to-treat analysis is important because it maintains the confounding control that randomization produces, whereas this is not the case if participants ultimately self-select into the treatment or comparison group. However, lack of adherence can cause bias, error, and confounding to occur. A good example of this "crossover" effect is an example of an RCT evaluating ibuprofen to treat altitude sickness, where 33% of those in the placebo group used ibuprofen during the study.[17]

Selection bias can occur through loss to follow-up in RCTs, similar to prospective cohort studies. If participants drop out of the study in a way that is related to both their exposure status and risk of outcome, then selection bias can occur. For this reason, RCTs need to closely follow up with their participants, and readers should be on the lookout for the reported follow-up rates in both treatment and control groups. Finally, external validity is often a concern. Participants who are willing to be randomized are not necessarily a random selection of the source population. The lack of representation of people who are non-White, non-urban, etc. in RCTs is well-documented.[18]

How do researchers select a study design?

Given all these possibilities, you are probably wondering how investigators choose which study design to use. Often there are multiple designs that could be used to address a specific research question. For example, Figure 4.2 describes how we could evaluate associations between intrauterine devices (IUDs) and ovarian cancer risk using four different study designs. An in-depth discussion of how to select a study design is beyond the scope of this book, but there are a couple of important pieces for us to consider that become relevant as we engage in a critical analysis of the literature.

First, research into a given question often starts with designs at the bottom of the hierarchy and then works its way up. For example, early evidence that cigarette smoking caused lung cancer came from case-series and case-control studies, followed by more definitive prospective cohort studies. The 1964 Report of the U.S. Surgeon General on

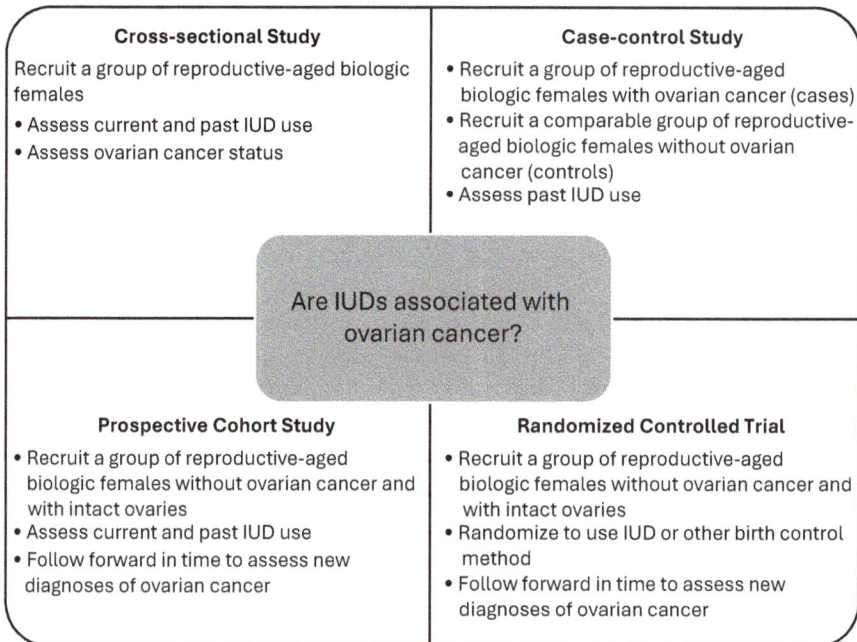

Cross-sectional Study

Recruit a group of reproductive-aged biologic females

- Assess current and past IUD use
- Assess ovarian cancer status

Case-control Study

- Recruit a group of reproductive-aged biologic females with ovarian cancer (cases)
- Recruit a comparable group of reproductive-aged biologic females without ovarian cancer (controls)
- Assess past IUD use

Are IUDs associated with ovarian cancer?

Prospective Cohort Study

- Recruit a group of reproductive-aged biologic females without ovarian cancer and with intact ovaries
- Assess current and past IUD use
- Follow forward in time to assess new diagnoses of ovarian cancer

Randomized Controlled Trial

- Recruit a group of reproductive-aged biologic females without ovarian cancer and with intact ovaries
- Randomize to use IUD or other birth control method
- Follow forward in time to assess new diagnoses of ovarian cancer

Figure 4.2 Oftentimes a single exposure–outcome relationship can be evaluated with multiple study designs, as in these examples of how to evaluate associations between intrauterine devices (IUDs) for birth control and ovarian cancer.

Smoking and Health provides a historical record of the accumulating evidence linking smoking to lung cancer, starting in 1939.[19] By the time the report was published, there was strong enough evidence accumulated that conducting an RCT would have been unethical.

Second, feasibility is very often the driving factor in the final choice of study design. Feasibility considerations often relate to the very finite resources of time and money—we may want to establish our own prospective cohort study and use a gold standard measurement of exposure, but the expense and logistics of such an undertaking are often so prohibitive that instead we perform a secondary analysis within an existing prospective cohort. We may decide that we would rather accept the limitations associated with an existing cohort's solid (but less than ideal) exposure assessment because otherwise we couldn't feasibly do the study at all.

Selecting the study design is a thoughtful decision made after careful consideration of the relative strengths, limitations, and feasibility of the different options. It often involves tradeoffs to maximize the strengths and minimize the limitations. Notice that I said "minimize" the limitations, not "eliminate" them. Epidemiologic studies always have limitations. Remember, we are working with humans, not laboratory animals. Even in an experimental design, we can never have complete control of all sources of variability, bias, confounding, and error. For this reason, *a single epidemiologic study is never definitive*. It is the accumulation of evidence across many similar studies over time that eventually gives us the answer.

Activities

Imagine that you are part of a research group seeking to evaluate associations between marijuana use and short-term memory loss among college students. As an initial step, you must select the study design to use.

1. Describe the strengths and limitations of each design under consideration:
   a) cross-sectional,
   b) case-control,
   c) prospective cohort, and
   d) randomized controlled trial.
2. Based on the strengths and limitations identified, which study design would you recommend to your research group? Why?

References

1. Pneumocystis Pneumonia — Los Angeles. Accessed January 9, 2024. https://www.cdc.gov/mmwr/preview/mmwrhtml/june_5.htm
2. Outbreak of West Nile-Like Viral Encephalitis – New York, 1999. Accessed January 9, 2024. https://www.cdc.gov/mmwr/preview/mmwrhtml/mm4838a1.htm
3. Crowe SJ, Bottichio L, Shade LN, et al. Shiga toxin–producing *E. coli* infections associated with flour. *N Engl J Med.* 2017;377(21):2036–2043. doi:10.1056/NEJMoa1615910
4. National Notifiable Diseases Surveillance System | CDC. March 15, 2024. Accessed July 11, 2024. https://www.cdc.gov/nndss/index.html
5. Vinikoor-Imler LC, Davis JA, Luben TJ. An ecologic analysis of county-level PM2.5 concentrations and lung cancer incidence and mortality. *Int J Environ Res Public Health.* 2011;8(6):1865–1871. doi:10.3390/ijerph8061865

6. Sasaki S, Horacsek M, Kesteloot H. An ecological study of the relationship between dietary fat intake and breast cancer mortality. *Prev Med.* 1993;22(2):187–202. doi:10.1006/pmed.1993.1016

7. Cao Y, Hou L, Wang W. Dietary total fat and fatty acids intake, serum fatty acids and risk of breast cancer: A meta-analysis of prospective cohort studies. *Int J Cancer.* 2016;138(8):1894–1904. doi:10.1002/ijc.29938

8. McGrath KG. An earlier age of breast cancer diagnosis related to more frequent use of antiperspirants/deodorants and underarm shaving. *Eur J Cancer Prev.* 2003;12(6):479–485. doi:10.1097/00008469-200312000-00006

9. American Cancer Society. *Breast Cancer Facts & Figures 2022–2024.* American Cancer Society, Inc; 2022.

10. Doll R, Hill AB. Smoking and lung cancer. *Br Med J.* 1953;1(4808):505. doi:10.1136/bmj.1.4808.505

11. SEER*Explorer: An interactive website for SEER cancer statistics [Internet]. *Surveillance Research Program, National Cancer Institute*; 2023 Apr 19. [updated: 2023 Nov 16; cited 2024 Jan 12]. Available from: https://seer.cancer.gov/statistics-network/explorer/. Data source(s): SEER Incidence Data, November 2022 Submission (1975–2020), SEER 22 registries (excluding Illinois and Massachusetts). Expected Survival Life Tables by Socio-Economic Standards. Accessed January 12, 2024.

12. Kilbo Edlund K, Andersson EM, Andersson M, et al. Occupational particle exposure and chronic kidney disease: A cohort study in Swedish construction workers. *Occup Environ Med.* 2024;81(5):238–243. doi:10.1136/oemed-2023-109371

13. Reeves KW, Díaz Santana M, Manson JE, et al. Urinary phthalate biomarker concentrations and postmenopausal breast cancer risk. *J Natl Cancer Inst.* 2019;111(10):1059–1067. doi:10.1093/jnci/djz002

14. Troeschel AN, Teras LR, Hodge JM, et al. A case-cohort study of per- and polyfluoroalkyl substance concentrations and incident prostate cancer in the cancer Prevention Study-II LifeLink cohort study. *Environ Res.* 2024;259:119560. doi:10.1016/j.envres.2024.119560

15. Winquist A, Hodge J, Diver WR, Teras L, Rodriguez J, Daniel J. Case-cohort study of the association between PFAS and selected cancers among participants in the American Cancer Society's Cancer Prevention II LifeLink cohort. *Environ Health Perspect.* 2023 Dec;131(12):127007. doi: 10.1289/EHP13174.

16. Mamluk L, Edwards HB, Savović J, et al. Low alcohol consumption and pregnancy and childhood outcomes: Time to change guidelines indicating apparently "safe" levels of alcohol during pregnancy? A systematic review and meta-analyses. *BMJ Open.* 2017;7(7):e015410. doi:10.1136/bmjopen-2016-015410

17. Gertsch JH, Corbett B, Holck PS, et al. Altitude sickness in climbers and efficacy of NSAIDs trial (ASCENT): Randomized, controlled trial of ibuprofen versus placebo for prevention of altitude illness. *Wilderness Environ Med.* 2012;23(4):307–315. doi:10.1016/j.wem.2012.08.001

18. Paskett ED, Reeves KW, McLaughlin JM, et al. Recruitment of minority and underserved populations in the United States: The Centers for Population Health and Health Disparities experience. *Contemp Clin Trials.* 2008;29(6):847–861. doi:10.1016/j.cct.2008.07.006

19. Smoking and Health. Reports of the Surgeon General - Profiles in Science. Accessed July 11, 2024. https://profiles.nlm.nih.gov/spotlight/nn/catalog/nlm:nlmuid-101584932X202-doc

CHAPTER 5

Who was in the study population?

It goes without saying that participants are an important part of any epidemiologic study. After all, if you don't have anyone to study, you won't have any results to report. Who is included, and who is not included, in a particular study has an important impact on the study's internal and external validity.

Often, investigators will set eligibility criteria for important reasons that can enhance the internal validity of the study (e.g., in a case-control study, cases are often required to meet strict diagnostic criteria). Sometimes, though, who ends up in the study is impacted by unwanted, and often unforeseen, forces. For example, research study populations may be at higher risk of the condition under study (e.g., individuals with a family history of a certain disease might be more likely to enroll in a study exploring risk factors for that disease). Study populations may end up being unrepresentative of the broader population for any number of reasons (e.g., a study enrolls participants from its local, urban population, while the vast majority of the state's residents live in rural areas). Sometimes these forces can cause bias and reduce the study's internal validity. Other times these forces are more of a nuisance—while they don't affect the internal validity of the results, they do raise concerns about generalizing the study's results to other populations (i.e., external validity).

As we read and critically analyze scientific articles, we need to carefully think through who was included, and who was not, and why. What processes impacted who ended up in the final study population? How representative is the final study population of the eligible population, of the population who was invited to participate, and of the general population? And, can we apply the results observed in this particular study to other populations?

In this chapter, we will explore ways in which selection of the study population can impact internal and external validity. We also will identify key issues to be on the lookout for as you read an epidemiologic article.

DOI: 10.4324/9781003637899-6

How were the participants recruited?

Epidemiologists often refer to multiple levels of participant selection (Figure 5.1). First, we can identify a **target population**, which is the population to which we wish to apply the study's results. Next, we identify a **source population**, which is the population we can access, screen for eligibility, and invite to participate. From the source population, we work to identify the **eligible population**, who are individuals from the source population meeting our prespecified inclusion and exclusion criteria. The **study population** is then comprised of those in the eligible population who enroll in the study. Within the study population, we often identify an **analytic sample**, which includes the participants contributing data to the analysis described in the manuscript.

As you read about a study's recruitment process, you should be paying attention to how individuals moved from the target population to the source population to the eligible population to the study population and, finally, to the analytic sample. Some important questions to ask: was the source population identified in a way that

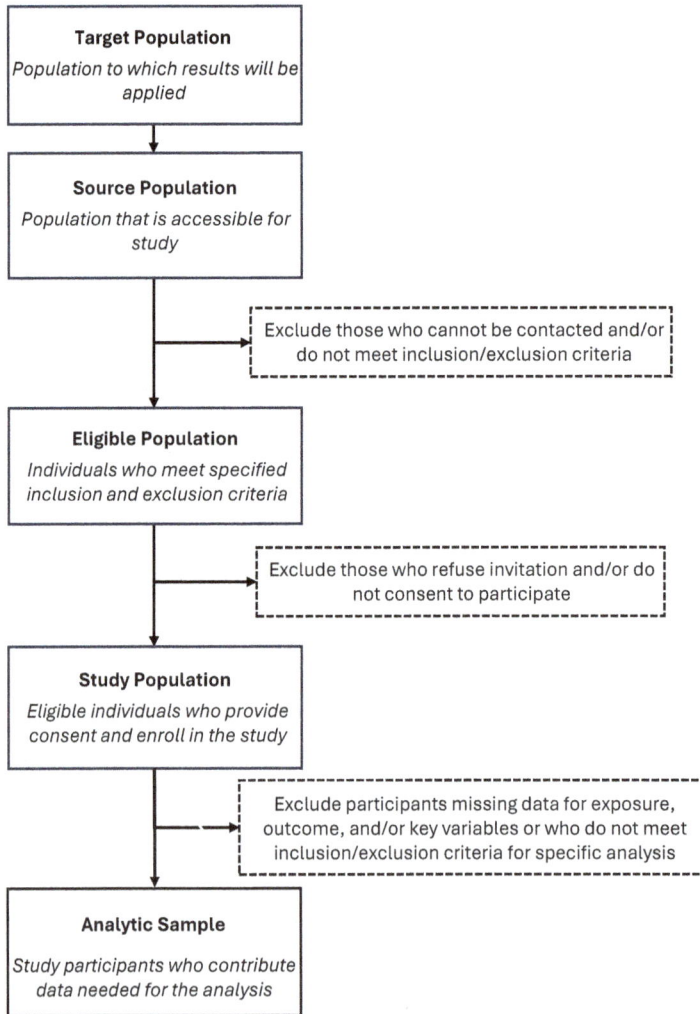

Figure 5.1 Selection of participants for a study involves identifying populations at multiple levels.

fully represents the target population? Was the eligible population reflective of the source population? Was the study population representative of the eligible population? Was the analytic sample representative of the study population?

The recruitment and screening procedures can impact who is (and is not) included at each level of selection. This is where those unwanted and unforeseen forces I mentioned earlier can creep in. Imagine that you want to conduct a case-control study of breast cancer risk factors, and you need to decide how to recruit controls. Because most breast cancer diagnoses are made from a screening mammogram, whether or not someone is diagnosed with breast cancer is directly related to their access to screening mammography, especially for disease in its earlier stages. In the U.S., access to cancer screening tests, as well as willingness to have the screening test even when access isn't an issue, can vary widely based on geographic location, race/ethnicity, health insurance status, and many other factors. If you decide to recruit controls from the nearby hospital's mammography clinic, you need to think through how these extraneous forces impact the representativeness of your control group in relation to the source and target populations. Furthermore, you also should consider whether the study population—cases and controls—has external validity, given the selection forces that make those who receive cancer screening different from those who do not.

Every epidemiologic article should provide a thorough description of the process used to recruit and enroll participants into the study. This description typically is given its own subsection within the Methods section, often coming first within that section. Researchers should specify the timeframe for recruitment, how potentially eligible participants were identified, and any inclusion or exclusion criteria that were used to determine eligibility. This description also should include the numbers of individuals at each step, starting from all those who were screened for eligibility and working down to how many ended up enrolling in the study and ultimately contributed to the analysis. Often, especially with complicated study designs, a flow chart is included showing the entire recruitment process (e.g., Figure 5.2).

Oftentimes, researchers will include a thorough description of the recruitment process in the first manuscript published using a study's data, which will be cited in subsequent manuscripts along with an abbreviated description. Some studies will publish an initial manuscript that only describes the recruitment processes and baseline characteristics of the study population (e.g., the Women's Health Initiative published an article describing their Observational Study cohort[2]). This is a common practice, and it should not raise red flags for you regarding the quality of the study. With journals limiting the word count of research manuscripts, researchers understandably choose to provide a brief overview of the recruitment process and cite prior publications for complete details (you can then identify those prior publications from the article's reference list and access them using PubMed). It does mean, though, that you will need to go back and read the prior publications' Methods sections to fully understand the recruitment process and consider its strengths and limitations as part of your critical analysis.

What were the specified eligibility criteria?

An important component of recruitment is specifying the eligibility criteria. Researchers will set eligibility criteria for participants prior to beginning their study or analysis. When you read the Methods section, the eligibility criteria should be clearly stated, well-justified, and applied equally across the study population groups.

```
┌─────────────────────────────┐
│  Females at risk for breast │
│           cancer            │
│                             │
│      Target Population       │
└─────────────────────────────┘
              │
              ▼
┌─────────────────────────────┐
│  Females living in western  │
│      Washington, USA        │
│                             │
│      Source Population       │
└─────────────────────────────┘
              │
              ▼
┌─────────────────────────────┐
│  White, English-speaking,   │
│       age 20-74 yrs         │
│                             │
│      Eligible Population      │
└─────────────────────────────┘
```

Cases: Diagnosed with Breast Cancer (Nov 1992-March 1995), identified through cancer registry
N=813 (78% of eligible)

Study Population: Cases

Controls: No history of breast cancer

N=793 (75% of eligible)

Study Population: Controls

Case providing data needed for analysis

N=683 (84% of study population)

Analytic Population: Cases

Controls providing data needed for analysis

N=697 (88% of study population)

Analytic Population: Controls

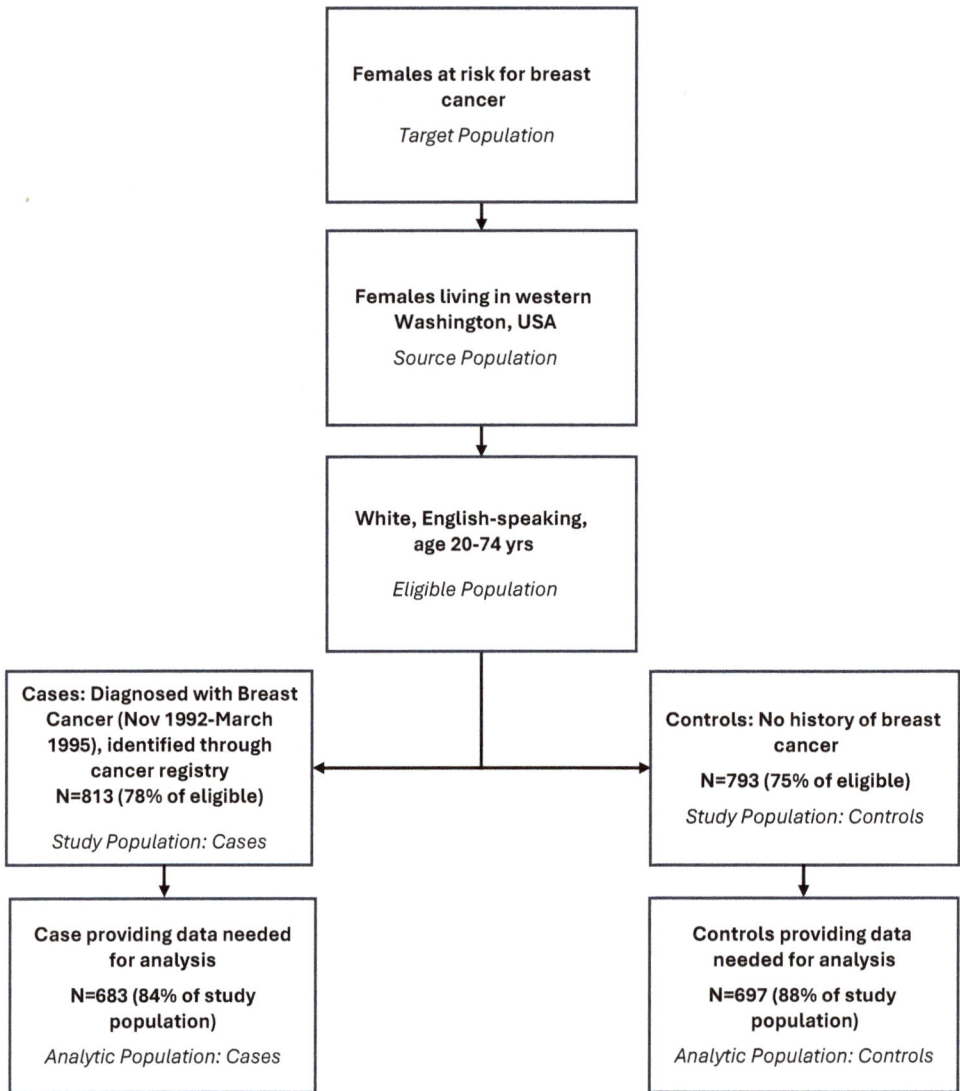

Figure 5.2 Example of a flow chart depicting the recruitment process from the Mirick et al. (2002)[1] study.

Eligibility criteria are chosen for important reasons, including ensuring that populations are at-risk for disease (e.g., excluding individuals without a prostate in a study of prostate cancer). Sometimes, eligibility criteria are set to restrict the population to a specific group of individuals who represent an important subgroup or to prevent confounding by an important factor (e.g., restricting to postmenopausal women to eliminate potential confounding by menstrual cycle timing). Very often, eligibility criteria are set for practical reasons related to carrying out the study (e.g., restricting to those who can read and/or speak English when translating services are not available). Sometimes, though, the eligibility criteria can result in a study population that is not representative of the source population (e.g., the source population includes a sizable proportion of non-English speakers/readers, and the distribution of exposure and disease in that population is different than that of the English-speaking/reading population).

Who ends up in the study population and analytic sample?

It won't surprise you to learn that not everyone who is eligible to join a study agrees to participate. When you read scientific articles, you need to pay attention to any differences between those who agreed to participate and those who did not.

One of the first things you will want to know is how many people who were eligible for the study ended up enrolling. This will be influenced by two general factors: (1) finding the eligible people and (2) having them agree to participate. In some cases, it may be easy to identify eligible participants without even having to contact them (e.g., finding all cases of influenza diagnosed at a hospital by searching medical records over a defined time period); in these situations, we can calculate a **participation rate** by reporting the percentage of eligible individuals who enroll in the study.

Sometimes, though, researchers are not able to enumerate all the eligible individuals because no such records exist (e.g., finding all individuals who have ever used illicit drugs within a given population). In these (more common) cases, a response rate is calculated instead. The **response rate** is the percentage of eligible individuals who were contacted and invited to participate who enrolled in the study. Note the subtle difference between the participation rate and the response rate: the participation rate measures enrollment among *all* eligible individuals, while the response rate measures enrollment among those eligible individuals who were successfully contacted and invited to participate.

The analytic sample is the subset of the study population that contributes data to the statistical analysis. Understanding who is included in the analytic sample and how they compare to the study population is also important. Sometimes the analytic sample may only include those who completed follow-up or who were not missing data on some key variable(s); these are understandable reasons for exclusion from the analysis, but they also can create opportunities for bias. As an extreme example, imagine that only the exposed participants with the outcome were missing data on an important confounder. If you excluded these participants from your analytic sample, you could end up with a biased result. We will explore this idea further in the next section of this chapter, as we dig deeper into selection bias and how it occurs in different study designs.

You may have noticed that "Table 1" in many articles presents a description of the study's analytic sample. Typically, this table reports descriptive statistics on key demographic factors (e.g., age, race/ethnicity, sex, and/or gender), as well as other factors that are relevant to the question under study (e.g., medical history, medication use, reproductive history, health behaviors). Case-control studies generally present these data stratified by case/control status, with statistical tests to identify differences between these groups. Prospective cohort and randomized controlled trials (RCTs) will report the same types of statistics and tests but instead grouping on exposure status. These tables are important to read carefully—they will give you a clear sense of who is (and is not) in the study population. As you will see shortly, inspecting these types of tables also can be helpful in evaluating whether selection bias is present.

What is selection bias?

Broadly speaking, **selection bias** occurs when the combination of exposure status and outcome status affects who is enrolled in the study (i.e., who is in the study population) and/or contributes data to the analysis (i.e., who is in the analytic sample). Whether the authors have reported a participation rate or a response rate, the basic idea is that the higher the percentage of eligible participants that enroll, the less likely it is that a selection bias is present and could impact the results. But even if 90% of eligible participants agree to enroll, there could still be a problem with the study population. Imagine, for example, if the 10% who refuse to enroll all belong to the same demographic group (e.g., all are non-English speakers) or all share the same risk factor (e.g., all are smokers). At a minimum, differences between the study population and the eligible population can make the study population lack representativeness of the source population. While high response rates reduce the likelihood of selection bias occurring, they don't fully eliminate the threat of selection bias. However, if enrolling in the study is jointly influenced by both the probability of exposure *and* the probability of outcome, we end up with selection bias (and a problem).

As an example (Figure 5.3), imagine a case-control study exploring whether COVID-19 vaccination (exposure) is associated with deep vein thrombosis (DVT; outcome). If cases who are vaccinated against COVID-19 are more likely to enroll in the study than those who are not vaccinated, the resulting study population would have an observed prevalence of exposure (COVID-19 vaccination) that is higher than the true prevalence of exposure among cases in the target population. If the same effect is present among the controls, then the resulting odds ratio would not be affected by selection bias. This is because the percentage of exposed cases who enroll and the percentage of exposed controls who enroll would be the same, keeping the ratio of exposed cases to exposed controls reflective of the background population (Study Population A). But, if there is some (known or unknown) reason that vaccination influences enrollment among cases but has no relationship to enrollment among controls (Study Population B), then we have a big problem. Selection bias would greatly impact our estimated association, perhaps causing us to incorrectly conclude that COVID-19 vaccination is positively associated with DVT.

You may be familiar with several specific examples of selection bias—sometimes the situation arises so commonly that it has its own name—but these examples still fall under the general umbrella of selection bias. Table 5.1 provides definitions and examples of some of the most common forms of selection bias. While case-control studies tend to be most susceptible to selection bias, selection bias can still happen in prospective cohort studies. Selection bias arises from the design of the study and the processes within it; we will go into detail about ways in which selection bias occurs in various study designs in the next few sections.

When is it not selection bias?

Students often mislabel situations where not all eligible cases and controls are enrolled or where a different percentage of controls are enrolled than cases (e.g., a study enrolls 75% of eligible cases but only 25% of eligible controls) as selection bias. We cannot automatically assume that selection bias is present in these situations; we must ask the question of whether exposure and outcome jointly affect the participation rates. Remember: it is not a selection bias if the exposure status of the cases or controls does

TARGET POPULATION (TRUTH)

	Cases	Controls
Vaccinated	500	500
Not Vaccinated	500	500
	1000	1000

True prevalence of exposure:
  Cases=50%
  Controls=50%
True OR= (500/500) / (500/500) = 1.0

A.Vaccination increases participation overall

STUDY POPULATION A (OBSERVED)

	Cases	Controls
Vaccinated	70	70
Not Vaccinated	30	30
	100	100

Observed prevalence of exposure:
  Cases=70%
  Controls=70%
Observed OR= (70/30) / (70/30) = 1.0

B.Vaccination increases participation among cases

STUDY POPULATION B (OBSERVED)

	Cases	Controls
Vaccinated	70	50
Not Vaccinated	30	50
	100	100

Observed prevalence of exposure:
  Cases=70%
  Controls=50%
Observed OR= (70/30) / (50/50) = 2.3

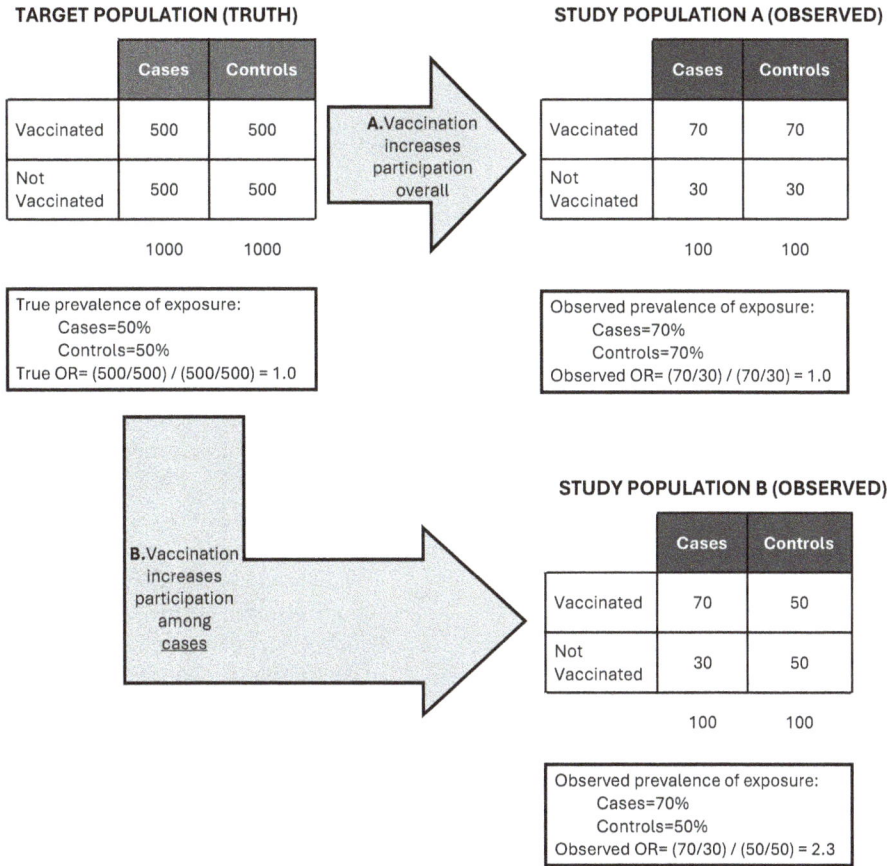

Figure 5.3 Illustrative example of selection bias in a case-control study. In Study Population A, exposed individuals are more likely to participate than unexposed individuals. Because participation rates by exposure status are not different between cases and controls, there is not a selection bias, and the estimated odds ratio reflects the true underlying odds ratio. In Study Population B, exposed cases are more likely to participate, which causes a selection bias resulting in an overestimate of the true odds ratio.

not influence their participation rates. These situations could raise concerns about sample size and/or representativeness to the target population, however.

Students also often get confused between selection bias and lack of representativeness of the study population. Let's consider an example (Figure 5.4) where we imagine conducting a study in a specific county, where 50% of the population identifies as non-Hispanic White. If we could, hypothetically, enroll everyone living in that county, we would calculate that exposure is associated with a two-times higher risk of outcome, meaning that exposure doubles the risk of the outcome.

Now, imagine that instead of enrolling everyone living in that county, we only enroll those residents who identify as non-Hispanic White (Study A in Figure 5.4). As a result, the study population does not reflect the racial/ethnic demographics of the county. We know that the study population does not match the demographic makeup of the county, but does this impact our results? If race/ethnicity is unrelated to the likelihood

Table 5.1 Common types of selection bias

Definition	Example
Volunteer or participation bias	
Individuals who agree to participate in research studies are often systematically different than those who refuse participation; when participation is jointly influenced by exposure and outcome status, selection bias occurs.	A study of predictors of colorectal cancer risk enrolls a higher proportion of individuals with a family history of colorectal cancer than is found in the general population, thus selectively including individuals with certain genetic mutations and a high risk of colorectal cancer and creating a selection bias when evaluating associations between genetic mutations and colorectal cancer risk.
Medical surveillance bias	
Individuals with certain exposures are often followed more closely and receive additional screening for certain medical conditions, making it appear that the exposure is associated with the disease.	A study evaluating associations between antidepressant use and hypertension reports a strong positive association, which is later determined to be a result of routine blood pressure screening among antidepressant users at their frequent clinical follow-up visits as compared to nonusers who only visit a health care provider and are screened for high blood pressure once per year.
Berksonian bias	
A bias specific to hospital-based case-control studies, where controls are recruited from patients who are hospitalized for conditions other than the disease under study. If the controls' conditions are also related to the exposure, the association between exposure and the disease under study will be underestimated.	A case-control study exploring whether coffee consumption is related to lung cancer risk enrolls cases having surgery and controls admitted to the same hospital for treatment of ulcers; because individuals with ulcers are less likely to drink coffee than the general population, there appears to be a positive association between coffee and lung cancer risk.
Healthy worker effect	
A bias specific to occupational studies, where cases/exposed are workers in a specific industry or at a specific employer. Because those who are able to work are generally healthier than those who are not able to work, selecting a comparison group (controls/unexposed) that is not restricted to workers can result in selection bias.	A study of glioblastoma among employees at an industrial plant reported similar incidence rates to the overall state population, yet elevated rates when comparing exposed workers to non-exposed workers.

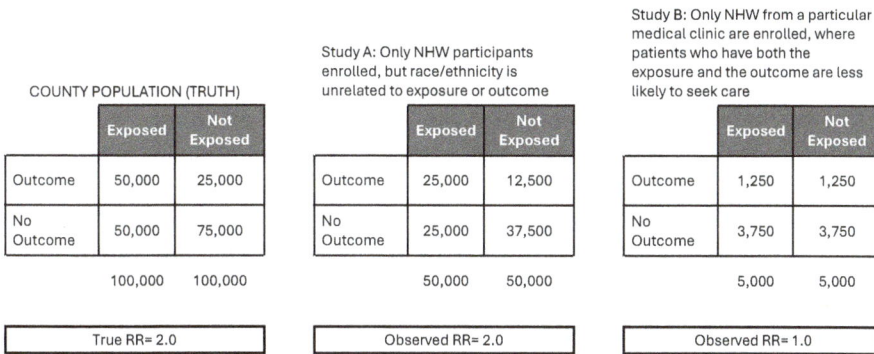

Figure 5.4 Illustration of how a "highly selected" population doesn't necessarily create selection bias.

of having the exposure and the outcome, we would still arrive at the correct conclusion: having the exposure doubles the risk of the outcome. While this will raise concerns about the external validity of the study's results (more about external validity soon), this is not a selection bias.

On the other hand, what if the participants' exposure status *and* their outcome status make them more (or less) likely to enroll? Imagine that instead our study is conducted by enrolling only non-Hispanic White individuals from a particular medical clinic, where the patients who are exposed and have the outcome are underrepresented (perhaps because they have more severe disease and end up seeking care elsewhere); this is Study B in Figure 5.4. Because selection into Study B is related to *both* exposure and outcome status, a selection bias is present. The selection bias, in this example, causes the observed relative risk (RR) to be an underestimate of the true RR, and Study B would (incorrectly) conclude that there is no association between exposure and outcome.

The above situations may seem unrealistic, but epidemiological studies are full of what could be described as "highly selected" populations. Famous examples of highly selected cohorts include the Framingham Heart Study (which initially enrolled only males living in a single, predominantly non-Hispanic White, community) and the Nurses' Health Studies (which enrolled only female registered nurses, a profession that was primarily non-Hispanic White at the time the initial study began). The fact that these studies included participants from a very specific segment of the population does not necessarily mean that the associations they estimated between exposure and outcome are affected by selection bias. But, it does mean that you would be right to question whether the results apply to demographics not represented within the study population. This is our old friend external validity, which we will come back to shortly.

How does selection bias typically happen in a case-control study?

Generally speaking, if there is going to be an issue with the study population in a case-control study, it tends to be with how the controls are selected. This is not to say that there can't (or won't) be issues with selecting cases, but recruiting healthy people to a study is typically far more difficult than recruiting those with the outcome under study. The goal in recruiting controls, of course, is to find a group of unaffected individuals who accurately reflect the exposure prevalence in the target population and who *would be* identified as a case in the study if they were diagnosed with the disease. But this is easier said than done. When reading an epidemiologic study, you need to carefully interrogate how both groups (cases and controls) were recruited and think about whether their exposure status might have made them more (or less) likely to be identified and enrolled.

As described above, if exposure somehow affects the likelihood of enrollment in one group (cases or controls) but not the other, then selection bias occurs. An important note is that, because selection bias relates to the exposure, a case-control study that assessed multiple exposures could have a selection bias associated with one exposure, but not another. Imagine a case-control study exploring risk factors for birth defects, with the two main factors of interest being: (1) concentrations of per-fluoroalkyl substances (PFAS) in drinking water and (2) substance use during pregnancy (Figure 5.5). Because people often do not know whether PFAS are present in their drinking water (let alone the exact concentrations), you could expect that PFAS concentrations in drinking water did not affect participation rates among cases or controls. If cases with substance use during pregnancy are less likely to enroll than controls with substance use *and* are less likely to enroll than cases without substance use, then the prevalence of substance use among enrolled cases no longer reflects the true prevalence of substance use in the target population. Here, substance use during pregnancy *did* affect participation rates, but only among the cases. As a result, there is selection bias.

This issue of selection bias being related to a specific exposure is especially important to think about in secondary analyses of data from case-control studies. It may be that there is no selection bias in relation to the original exposure under study, but selection bias could arise if the exposure under study in the secondary analysis influenced participation.

How does selection bias typically happen in a prospective cohort or randomized controlled trial?

Remember when I said that selection bias happens when exposure status and outcome status together impact participation in the study? Given that outcome status is not yet known in prospective designs (including prospective cohort studies and RCTs), these types of studies are far less prone to selection bias. This is good news, indeed.

But, don't think that you can just forget all about selection bias when you are critically analyzing a prospective study or RCT. In fact, because the ways that selection bias occurs in these designs are a bit sneakier, you might need to pay even more attention to looking for opportunities for selection bias in these designs. In these types of studies, selection bias can occur from: (1) differential loss to follow-up or (2) missing data. Generally speaking, the smaller the number of participants who are left out of the analytic sample due to loss to follow-up or missing data, the lower the chances that selection bias would affect the results.

Loss to follow-up is a catch-all phrase for when participants fail to complete the study. As a result, investigators don't know whether or not they experienced the outcome during the study period. Common reasons for loss to follow-up include moving, withdrawing from the study, or death. Oftentimes these reasons have no relationship

A.

TARGET POPULATION (TRUTH)

	Cases	Controls
High PFAS	1250	1000
Low PFAS	1250	1500
	2500	2500

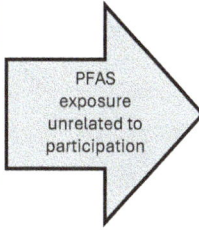

PFAS exposure unrelated to participation

STUDY POPULATION (OBSERVED)

	Cases	Controls
High PFAS	125	100
Low PFAS	125	150
	250	250

True prevalence of high PFAS exposure:
Cases=50%
Controls=40%
True OR = (1250/1250) / (1000/1500) = 1.5

Observed prevalence of high PFAS exposure:
Cases=50%
Controls=40%
Observed OR= (125/125) / (100/150) = 1.5

B.

TARGET POPULATION (TRUTH)

	Cases	Controls
Substance use	1500	500
No substance use	1000	2000
	2500	2500

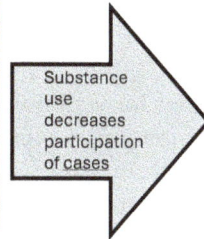

Substance use decreases participation of cases

STUDY POPULATION (OBSERVED)

	Cases	Controls
Substance use	75	50
No substance use	175	200
	250	250

True prevalence of substance use:
Cases=60%
Controls=20%
True OR = (1500/1000) / (500/2000) = 6.0

Observed prevalence of substance use:
Cases=30%
Controls=20%
Observed OR= (75/175) / (50/200) = 1.7

Figure 5.5 Selection bias occurs when inclusion in a study is related to both prevalence of exposure and risk of outcome. In Panel A, there is no relationship between exposure to PFAS and outcome status, resulting in an unbiased estimate of the odds ratio. However, in Panel B, cases with exposure to substance use during pregnancy are less likely to participate compared to other groups, resulting in a biased estimation of the odds ratio.

to the exposure or outcome under study. But, when they do, selection bias can occur. Imagine a prospective cohort study evaluating whether physical activity is related to risk of diabetes (Figure 5.6). You can imagine that participants who are the least physically active might also experience health challenges that cause them to be lost to follow-up and that these same individuals are those with the highest actual risk of diabetes. As a result, the analytic sample includes an under-representation of those with low physical activity who end up being diagnosed with diabetes.

STUDY POPULATION (TRUTH)

	High Physical Activity	Low Physical Activity
Diabetes	100	200
No Diabetes	900	800
	1000	1000

90% follow-up <u>except</u> for those with low PA and high diabetes risk, where follow-up is only 50%

ANALYTIC DATASET (OBSERVED)

	High Physical Activity	Low Physical Activity
Diabetes	90	100
No Diabetes	810	720
	900	820

True RR= (100/1000) / (200/1000) = 0.5

Observed RR= (90/900) / (100/820) = 0.8

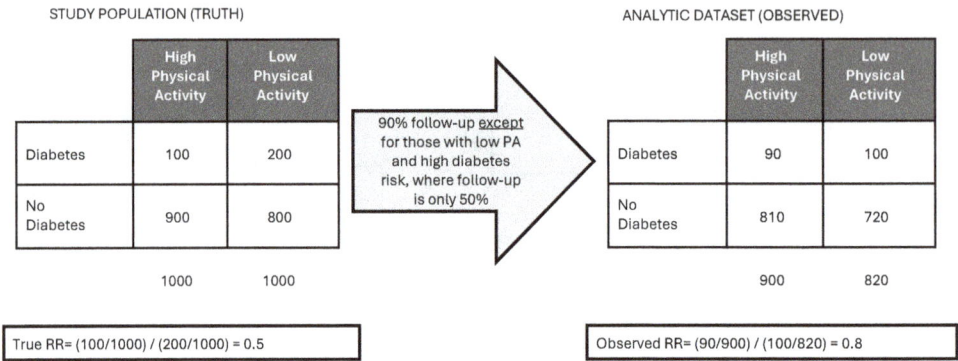

Figure 5.6 In prospective studies, selection bias may occur through differential loss to follow-up, such that there is a difference in follow-up that is related to both exposure status and potential for outcome.

Missing data present a similar scenario. Most studies will have some level of missing data, and missing data create a whole list of problems, including negative impacts on statistical power (more to come on that issue in Chapter 8). But when the pattern of missingness is related to both exposure and outcome status, it also can create a selection bias if only those without missing data are included in the analytic sample (often referred to as a "complete-case analysis").

As a way of exploring the potential for selection bias in prospective studies, it is often useful to compare the joint distribution of exposure and outcome status between those participants included in the final analytic sample and those participants who were excluded due to missing data or loss to follow-up. You would ask, does the prevalence of exposure (or, the incidence of outcome) differ between those in the analytic sample and those who were excluded? Of course, this type of exploration won't be possible if the missing data are in the exposure or outcome.

How do I figure out if selection bias is present in a study?

Now that you understand what selection bias is and how it typically rears its ugly head in different study designs, let's describe approaches for identifying whether it is likely to be present as you read epidemiologic studies.

Before we go any further, I need to make a very important disclaimer: *there is not a definitive test for selection bias!* Instead, you will explore possibilities and make a reasoned judgment as to the probability of bias and the potential level of distortion. Thinking back to the buckets from Chapter 3, you will ask: is selection bias a minor concern, moderate concern, or major concern?

Some of these approaches may be more or less feasible, depending on the article. Sometimes, the authors will have done the work for you—you might see that they have included some of these analyses within their results or that they have provided this type of evidence within their Discussion section. Other times, you might be able to do the analysis on your own, either by accessing their data (easier for publicly available data) or by making comparisons using external data sources (e.g., using data collected on the target population by government public health agencies). In many cases, though, you can only think through hypothetical scenarios and weigh the likelihood that these scenarios would have caused a selection bias to have occurred.

Below is an overview of approaches you can use to assess the likelihood of selection bias when you are critically analyzing an epidemiologic study. For readers who want a far more in-depth examination, I refer you to a textbook by Savitz and Wellenius,[3] which provides a detailed discussion of this topic, including excellent examples. *Remember that you are never going to have definitive "yes" or "no" answer as to the presence (or absence) of selection bias; your goal is rather to consider the likelihood that selection bias is present.* The following approaches, then, will either reassure you or cause you concern.

- *Compare the participants who were included in the study and/or analysis to those who were not included.* Do the participants who were lost to follow-up differ from those who were not (e.g., by exposure status)? Are those who were missing data different from those who were not? Are there important differences between those who were (or may have been) eligible to participate and did not enroll and those who did enroll? Oftentimes, investigators will be able to collect very basic information on all those who were offered enrollment (e.g., age, sex, race/ethnicity, disease stage) and can perform statistical tests to identify differences between those who enrolled and those who did not. However, it is not always possible to collect such information on nonparticipants.
- *Consider whether there are important features of how the outcome is diagnosed that might cause the cases and controls to not be comparable.* This is where you need to have some knowledge about the diagnostic process for the outcome under study. Is it something that often goes undetected? Does diagnosis involve specialized medical tests? Then, consider whether everyone in the source population has equal access to, and utilization of, these diagnostic processes. For example, patients with a high body mass index (BMI) might be routinely tested for diabetes, whereas those with underweight or normal-range BMI might not be. If the study enrolls diabetes cases based on self-report, then, the case group would include only those who had been tested. The enrolled case group would be overrepresented by those in the overweight/obese BMI ranges and not be appropriately representative of all individuals who truly have diabetes (but are unaware due to lack of testing).
- *Examine patterns of loss to follow-up and of missing data.* Are these issues more (or less) common among the exposed and/or those with the outcome? Are there other important groups that have higher rates of missing data or loss to follow-up (e.g., defined by age, race/ethnicity, and socioeconomic status) and so are excluded from the analytic sample, even though they enrolled in the study? Remember, the higher the follow-up rates and/or the lower the amount of missing data, the more reassured we are that the impact of selection bias, if present, would be minimized.
- *Compare the prevalence of the exposure among the control group (or of the study population in a prospective cohort study) to that of the target population.* This is where data from public health agencies such as the U.S. Centers for Disease Control and Prevention and state and local health departments can be very helpful. For example, if BMI is our primary exposure in a diabetes case-control study, we might compare the distribution of BMI in the control group to that of the local, state, and/or national population.

■ *Compare the risk of outcome among the unexposed to that in the target population.* Recall that the unexposed group is meant to reflect the background risk of disease in the population, so if the risk among the unexposed is much higher (or much lower) for an outcome than the target population, this could be cause for concern. You would then want to look further to see what factors, including the exposure of interest, might have impacted participation among eligible controls.

■ *Explore whether expected associations between the exposure and other characteristics are observed in the study population, especially among the controls in a case-control study.* Seeing expected patterns can be reassuring, while *not* seeing those patterns raises red flags about the potential for selection bias. For example, if you observe that BMI is positively associated with reported physical activity among the controls (i.e., heavier people exercised more), then you should wonder if something is amiss that might have affected participation in the study based on BMI and outcome status.

■ *Explore whether known risk factors for the outcome are associated with the outcome within the study population.* For example, it is well-established that family history of diabetes is positively associated with diabetes risk. A study that does not demonstrate this positive association, or perhaps even shows the opposite association, should raise a red flag for you about whether a selection bias could be present.

What is external validity?

External validity refers to the ability of a study's results to be applied to populations beyond those included in the study. Most students are taught three things about external validity: (1) it means "generalizability," (2) it is determined by how representative the study population is of other populations, and (3) a study cannot be externally valid if it is not internally valid. Each of these things is true, and they each seem to make sense to students.

Where students struggle, though, is in thinking deeply about whether a study is, or is not, externally valid. Many students default to an approach of "this study only includes (or, perhaps, excludes) this particular group of people defined by age/race/geographic location; therefore, it has no external validity." This is a major oversimplification, however.

Instead, you must consider whether the mechanism(s) that cause the exposure to lead to the outcome would truly differ in groups of another age/race/geographic location. Sometimes, the answer is no. For example, a study conducted in a population recruited from Massachusetts that observed an association between nonsteroidal anti-inflammatory drug (NSAID) use and prevention of breast cancer is very likely to have external validity to populations in other U.S. states. This is because it is unlikely that the biological mechanisms that cause NSAIDs to reduce breast cancer risk would be impacted by one's state of residence.

However, if the same study of NSAIDs and breast cancer included only White women, we would rightly question whether the results would have external validity to Black women. This is because we know that Black women tend to be diagnosed with more aggressive forms of breast cancer and have different pathologic subtypes than White women.[4] There is evidence that the biology of the disease differs between these two population groups. As a result, we cannot assume that the association between NSAIDs and breast cancer would be equivalent for White women and Black women. In other words, the results may not be generalizable to non-White populations.

Just like selection bias, external validity is not a "yes" or "no" question. Instead, we are looking for evidence that either reassures us or causes us concern. There is one situation, though, where you can definitely say that the study is *not* externally valid. Can you guess when? That's right—when you have determined that the study is not *internally* valid.

So, how do you evaluate external validity, assuming you have already decided that the study has at least a reasonable degree of internal validity (based on our thorough assessment of the study population and the other threats to internal validity that we will cover in the next several chapters)? You need to go back to your understanding of the recruitment process and how participants were identified and invited to participate, and then how many of them enrolled and contributed to the analysis. Are there important groups (demographic or otherwise) that are not included at all or that are underrepresented? Did response rates vary based on some key factor(s) such that important groups are not represented in sufficient numbers? Is there reason to believe that the biological mechanisms linking exposure to outcome would vary based on these factors? Are there known or hypothesized interactions between these factors and the exposure?

An important final comment is to remember that scientific understanding of physiological processes is constantly changing, yet it is always incomplete. Because scientists don't fully understand all the processes that may link exposure to the outcome, you cannot assume that, for example, a result observed in White men would be applicable to Hispanic men, Black men, Asian men, and so on. It *might* have external validity to those populations, but it also might not. Replicating results in other populations is important, as that will be the true test of external validity.

STAR in action: examining the study population in Mirick et al.

Table 5.2 shows how the STAR template can be used to critically evaluate the study population of the Mirick article, considering all the aspects described in this chapter.

Although few details regarding recruitment are provided in this article, the authors reference an earlier publication describing recruitment in detail. Briefly, the study included White, English-speaking females living in western Washington state between the ages of 20 and 74 at the time of recruitment from November 1992 through March 1995. Eligibility criteria were the same for cases and controls, with the exception that cases recently had been diagnosed with breast cancer. Controls were identified using random-digit dialing and were frequency matched to cases in 5-year age groups. Because participants were recruited from the same source population, with appropriate and equivalent eligibility criteria, and with high response rates (78% cases, 75% controls), there is minimal concern for selection bias.

One limitation, however, is that all participants self-identified as White. Given known differences in breast cancer incidence rates and the distribution of breast cancer subtypes across racial/ethnic groups, we cannot assume that findings in this all-White population will necessarily be generalizable to other racial/ethnic groups.

Table 5.2 Completed STAR template Section 2: "Study Population" for Mirick et al. (2002)[1]

2. Study population	
Describe (i.e., report just the facts described in the article)	Critique (i.e., think through strengths/ limitations of the methods and results, address the key questions listed, and add additional comments as needed)
What is the source population? Be specific— include geographic region, calendar time, age, race, ethnicity, sex, etc.	Is this an appropriate population in which to address the stated objective/purpose? Why or why not?
Target population: females in the U.S. Source population: White English-speaking females from western Washington State from November 1992 to March 1995 ages of 20–74.	Restricting to western part of Washington State might not make the results generalizable to the rest of the U.S. or world. As that geographic area might not be as diverse as other populations or lack access to health care, etc. Also, they restricted their participants to White females, which does not necessarily make these results generalizable to other diverse populations. Note that few details are given in this article; readers are referred to prior publication.
What eligibility criteria were specified?	Are these criteria appropriate? Why or why not?
(refer to prior publication cited by authors) Female, White, English-speaking, living in western Washington state Cases were diagnosed with breast cancer from November 1992 to March 1995 and 20–74 years old at age of diagnosis. Controls were women without breast cancer from the source population that produced cases.	Yes, eligibility criteria are same for cases and controls (except for disease); criteria ensure cases are truly cases.
How were participants selected and/or recruited?	Could the study results have been affected by selection bias? Did the method of subject selection differ between comparison groups (i.e., differential loss to follow-up in exposed compared to unexposed in a cohort study; differential selection of cases compared to non-cases in a case-control study)?
Cases were women between the ages of 20–74 who were diagnosed with breast cancer from November 1992 to March 1995; identified from a cancer registry; N = 813 cases Controls identified through random-digit dialing (a common and appropriate approach at the time of the study) from the same source population as the cases; matched in 5-year age group; N = 793 controls	No; controls came from the same source population as the cases and were frequency-matched by 5-year age groups. They also note that if multiple controls were eligible at one household, they randomly selected one.

(Continued)

Table 5.2 (*Continued*)

2. *Study population*

	Were response/participation rates sufficient? Describe direction, magnitude, and likelihood.
	Minimal potential for selection bias since cases and controls selected from the same source population using the same eligibility criteria; unlikely that exposure status affected the probability of being selected as case or control.
	Response rates were high and were similar between cases (78%) and controls (75%), further minimizing selection bias.
	To what larger population may the results of this study be generalized (e.g., the source population, additional groups)? If you include groups beyond the source population, justify why. If you think results couldn't be applied to certain groups, justify why.
	Generalizable to White women ages 20–74 in Washington State. Likely also generalizable to White women in U.S.
	May not be generalizable to other countries or other racial/ethnic groups in the U.S.
	What other strengths and/or limitations do you note?
	Cases were incident (reduces potential survival bias) and identified through cancer registry (reduces misclassification)
	Unclear how controls were verified to not have breast cancer, which could lead to outcome misclassification

Activities

Find a recently published observational study or randomized controlled trial on a topic of interest to you. You might consider using the same article you read for the Activities from Chapter 3.

1. Describe the levels of participant selection, identifying the: target population, source population, eligible population, study population, and analytic population. Create a flow chart (similar to Figure 5.2) that shows the complete selection process, noting eligibility criteria and the numbers included or excluded at each step.

2. Complete Section 2 of the STAR template for this article to describe how participants were recruited and selected and evaluate the potential for selection bias as
well as the potential impact on external validity.
3. If you were to perform a similar study, how might you make different choices
regarding participant selection to improve the study's internal and external validity?

References

1. Mirick DK, Davis S, Thomas DB. Antiperspirant use and the risk of breast cancer. *J Natl Cancer Inst.* 2002;94(20):1578–1580. doi:10.1093/jnci/94.20.1578
2. Langer RD, White E, Lewis CE, Kotchen JM, Hendrix SL, Trevisan M. The Women's Health Initiative Observational Study: Baseline characteristics of participants and reliability of baseline measures. *Ann Epidemiol.* 2003;13(9 Suppl):S107–S121.
3. Savitz DA, Wellenius GA. *Interpreting Epidemiologic Evidence: Connecting Research to Applications*, 2nd ed. Oxford University Press; 2016.
4. Giaquinto AN, Sung H, Miller KD, et al. Breast cancer statistics, 2022. *CA Cancer J Clin.* 2022;72(6):524–541. doi:10.3322/caac.21754

How was the exposure measured?

Most epidemiologic studies can be boiled down to studying the association between an exposure and an outcome. Defining and measuring these things, though, can be fairly complicated. In the next two chapters, we will take a closer look at how the approach used to measure the exposure (Chapter 6) and outcome (Chapter 7) can affect the internal validity of the study.

Often, there will be many options for defining and measuring a single exposure. Imagine that your research team is interested in studying the effects of antidepressant use (Table 6.1). You likely would discuss the strengths and limitations of several different approaches: self-report, pharmacy records, primary care provider records, and measuring blood metabolites. Your group might wonder, which is the best (i.e., the most valid) approach to use? Does one approach have a higher (or lower) probability of error than another? Which approach is the most feasible? What time period of exposure is the most relevant to measure? And, what exactly do we want to measure: ever use? current use? use of specific formulations? dosage? duration of use?

Exposure assessment can get complicated quickly. In this chapter, we will consider important issues that are relevant to assessing the exposure under study. You will learn to evaluate the potential for bias and error in the exposure assessment, and you will think through how such bias or error impacts the study's findings.

What do epidemiologists mean by "exposure" anyway?

Before we get too deep into exposure assessment, we first need to clarify what the "exposure" is. It will be hard for you to critically evaluate the exposure if you can't identify what it is. In general, epidemiologists phrase their research questions as whether "exposure" is associated with "outcome."

As reviewed in Chapter 2, the "exposure" in an epidemiologic study is the factor being evaluated for a potential association with the outcome of interest. An exposure could be any number of things: a treatment (e.g., a new drug or therapy), a physical

DOI: 10.4324/9781003637899-7

Table 6.1 There often are multiple approaches that could be used to measure a given exposure. For example, "antidepressant (AD) use" could be measured through self-report, through pharmacy records, through primary care provider records, or through measuring blood metabolites. Each approach has both strengths and limitations, and investigators weigh these as they select a measurement approach for their study

Approach for measuring antidepressant (AD) use	Strengths	Limitations
Self-report *Ask participants on a self- or interviewer-administered survey to report their current and previous AD use*	■ Participants are likely to know what they are taking currently ■ Participants can be asked to look at pill bottles to improve reporting of current use ■ Can give examples/names to aid recall of previous use ■ Can specifically assess what participants are taking (and not just what they have been prescribed and perhaps never took)	■ Potential inaccuracy in reporting, especially for previous use ■ Must specify a time period that is etiologically appropriate (e.g., current use would not be etiologically relevant in a case-control study)
Pharmacy records *Retrieve records from participants' pharmacies to identify dispensed prescriptions for ADs over an established time period*	■ No potential for errors due to participant recall ■ Can collect data on exact medication, dose, and duration of use	■ Participants may not have taken filled prescriptions ■ Participants may fill prescriptions at multiple pharmacies and/or switch pharmacies over time ■ Need to ensure pharmacies serve entire study base ■ Must specify a time period that is etiologically appropriate (e.g., current use would not be etiologically relevant in a case-control study) ■ Pharmacies may not have records going back to etiologic period ■ Abstracting data from pharmacy records can be resource-intensive ■ Potential for random error

(Continued)

Table 6.1 *(Continued)*

Approach for measuring antidepressant (AD) use	Strengths	Limitations
Primary Care Provider (PCP) records *Retrieve medical records from participants' PCPs to identify prescriptions written for ADs and/or use of ADs recorded in medical record*	■ No potential for errors due to participant recall ■ Can collect data on exact medication, dose, and duration of use	■ Participants may have been given prescriptions from other providers that are not documented in PCP records ■ Participants may not have filled or taken prescriptions as directed ■ Must specify a time period that is etiologically appropriate (e.g., current use would not be etiologically relevant in a case-control study) ■ PCP may not have records going back to etiologic period ■ Abstracting data from PCP records can be resource-intensive ■ Potential for random error
Blood metabolites *Take a blood sample from participants and use a laboratory assay to measure metabolites of common Ads*	■ Objective measurement that is not susceptible to recall bias or other inaccuracies in reporting and/or records	■ Blood samples are considered moderately invasive and some participants may not provide consent ■ Only assesses current and very recent AD use, which may not be etiologically relevant ■ Requires clinic visit and research staff to obtain blood sample ■ Laboratory measurement incurs additional costs Potential for random error

measurement (e.g., body weight, blood pressure), a demographic characteristic (e.g., age, race, ethnicity), a behavior (e.g., smoking, physical activity), a social characteristic (e.g., political affiliation, sexual orientation)—the list could go on.

Sometimes, the same factor could be studied as an exposure in one study yet studied as the outcome in another. For example, you could evaluate what factors predict the risk of depression (as an outcome), and you also could explore whether depression (as an exposure) predicts the risk of other outcomes.

How was the exposure measured in the study?

The best measure of exposure is the one that comes closest to measuring the true value of the exposure at a time when it could have impacted the development of the outcome.

Exposures can be measured in a seemingly infinite number of ways. One exposure can even have many different approaches to its measurement, and those approaches may have a broad range in their validity. Some of the most common approaches for measuring a particular exposure include: (1) self-reporting presence or absence of exposure, (2) administering an established questionnaire or scale, (3) reviewing medical or other existing records, and (4) performing a physical or biological measurement. So, which of these approaches is the "best" one? And, how do you define what we mean by "best"?

As you might guess, each of these approaches comes with its own set of strengths and limitations. Often investigators must make tradeoffs as they select an approach for measuring the exposure, balancing practical concerns (e.g., finances, burden on participants) with the potential for bias and error.

Let's consider each general approach in turn, paying close attention to the features of these approaches that might make them closer to or farther from the "best" measurement approach, including questions of feasibility.

Self-report

Many exposures can be measured fairly accurately by simply asking the participants about their exposure history. Important strengths of self-report include that it is often the most feasible approach, as it is typically the fastest and least expensive approach. Whether these strengths outweigh the limitations, though, will depend on the particular exposure being measured. People can often accurately report exposures that are (a) occurring at the time of the report or in the very recent past, (b) not stigmatizing, and (c) known to them.

For example, adult participants in a prospective cohort study could likely self-report how many glasses of milk they currently drink each day with a high degree of accuracy. But if you instead wanted to know how many glasses of milk they drank each day as a *child*, these same participants might have difficulty remembering, and the accuracy of their responses would decrease.

Or, imagine that instead of asking about milk, you were interested in alcohol. Participants might underreport their alcohol consumption, especially at the highest levels and/or during certain time periods (e.g., childhood, pregnancy), due to concerns about social stigma.

Last, imagine that you wanted to know about participants' exposure to bisphenol-A (BPA), a chemical that is often found in plastic bottles, like those that are used to package gallons of milk. Asking participants about their exposure to BPA, though, would not be very useful, because most consumers have no idea whether or not they have been exposed to BPA through food packaging or the many other consumer products that often contain this chemical. Asking participants about how often they consume foods packaged in plastic might get you close, but the accuracy of that approach to measuring BPA exposure would still be quite poor.

Often, self-reports are done either by having participants complete a questionnaire themselves or by interviewing them. Self-administered questionnaires are typically less expensive to implement, as they require fewer research staff. They are most appropriate for questions that are straightforward to ask and answer, as no one is available to provide additional clarification to participants who don't understand the questions. Many times, self-administered questionnaires are used to ask about particularly sensitive topics (e.g., substance use, sexual history); participants may be more likely to accurately report these exposures when they can remain anonymous and/or can avoid having to verbally provide this information to another person.

Sometimes, though, studies use interviewers to assess participants' exposure history. While interviewers can promote the validity of exposure assessment in many ways (e.g., allowing for more complicated questions than could be asked on a self-administered questionnaire), they can also open the possibility for interviewer bias in case-control studies.

Interviewer bias occurs when the interviewer probes more deeply into the exposure of cases than controls (or vice versa). Imagine that an interviewer, aware of the study hypothesis that pesticide use causes Parkinson's disease, asks both cases and controls the same questions on the script but then goes off-script only with the cases, probing them with different pesticide names and possible times in their lives when they may have come into contact with them. It would be possible, in that scenario, that the exposure reporting among the cases might be different from controls because they had been asked more detailed questions, not because their actual exposure histories were truly different. For this reason, it is important that any investigators involved in assessing exposure status in a case-control study are unaware of the disease status of all participants (this is often referred to as "masking" or "blinding") and that they are trained to not deviate from the interviewer script.

Administering an established questionnaire or scale

Many exposures are measured so often that researchers have established, and validated, approaches to measuring them through questionnaires or scales. If such a questionnaire or scale exists, it can be very helpful to use it. You can think of using an established questionnaire or scale as a form of self-report, but one that can involve more complicated reporting. For example, instead of asking "have you felt depressed in the past two weeks?" to measure depressive symptoms, you could use a validated scale that asks individuals about common symptoms of depression and then uses a scoring system to identify those with significant depressive symptoms. Using established questionnaires or scales has at least two key benefits. First, independent validation provides confidence that the tool accurately measures the desired exposure. Second, using the standard tool facilitates comparison across populations and studies.

For example, the short form 36 health survey questionnaire (SF-36) has been validated for evaluating health-related quality of life in many populations, including primary care patients,[1] stroke patients,[2] and elderly participants,[3] as well as in translation to other languages including Arabic[4] and Spanish.[5]

Reviewing medical or other existing records

Some exposures might be recorded routinely in records or databases. For example, weight is typically measured and recorded every time a patient visits a medical provider. Or, a school might maintain records of students' grades that could be accessed and used to measure academic performance as an exposure in a research study. An important advantage of using these types of records is that they already exist. In other words, researchers don't need to collect the data themselves, meaning that the exposure data can often be obtained more quickly and at a lower overall cost. Further advantages include that these records are not subject to poor memory or to wishful thinking.

However, there are important limitations to consider as well. First, you need to recognize that such records often were not collected for the purpose of a research study. As a result, they can often be incomplete and lead to a missing data problem. And, the completeness of those records might even relate to whether or not someone has the outcome being studied, or another outcome, which could lead to bias. For example, someone with a chronic medical condition would likely be visiting their medical provider more frequently than someone without a chronic medical condition; therefore, weight measurements also would occur more frequently for someone with, versus without, a chronic disease.

Also, you need to consider what aspects of the exposure are important and how well those are measured. Imagine that a study is interested in exploring effects related to a particular medication. An advantage of using medical records or pharmacy records is that researchers could access accurate information on the medication name, dosage, and even duration of use. But even these records have limitations. Medical records could tell you that a medication was prescribed, but not whether the patient actually filled the prescription. Pharmacy records could tell you whether the prescription was filled, but not whether the participant took the medication as prescribed. Again, nothing in epidemiology is ever perfect!

Last, it can be challenging to retrieve medical or other records for all participants, unless the availability of such records is somehow built into the recruitment process. For example, researchers might conduct a study using members of a specific health insurance plan, thus ensuring access to medical claims information on all participants. On the other hand, if participant medical records are needed and those participants all have different health care providers, it will be more difficult to retrieve those records from multiple clinics. And, some participants may not consent to allowing investigators to access their medical records, which would lead to missing data. You also should recognize that, although medical records are considered the gold standard, they too are created by humans, and so they can still have some level of error.

Performing a physical or biological test

Many exposures can be measured by doing either a routine or a specialized test. For example, participants' height and weight can easily be measured in a medical or research study clinic using their standard equipment. These types of objective measurements have a lot of advantages, as they eliminate errors due to participant recall or general errors in self-reporting.

However, even seemingly objective measurements can have opportunities for error. It is important to ensure that any instruments used for physical measurements are well-calibrated. This is especially important in multicenter studies, where different pieces of equipment will be used to measure the exposure; ensuring that the different pieces of equipment are calibrated with one another is important for ensuring apples-to-apples comparisons among the participants.

Another important consideration is the experience of the person performing the assessment. Some measurements might be easily performed (e.g., height and weight), while others may require specialized training and experience (e.g., neurological testing).

Additionally, in case-control studies, it is important that whoever is performing the exposure measurements is masked to the outcome status of the participants. In the context of case-control studies, an additional important issue is that the assessment measures physical/biological characteristics *after* the outcome has occurred. This timing generates significant temporality concerns (and, concerns about whether the measured characteristics were impacted by the outcome). I should note, though, that this concern does not apply to *nested* case-control studies, where the exposure assessment is made using samples and/or data collected well before the occurrence of the outcome.

For measurements made in a laboratory using biological samples such as blood or urine, there are additional issues you should consider. First, concentrations of some biological substances (e.g., glucose) can vary substantially depending on the time of day the sample is taken and whether or not the participant was fasting. Some substances (e.g., hormones) might have variability related to menstrual cycle stage. Understanding the conditions under which the samples were taken relative to known biologic variation is highly important for evaluating the accuracy of the exposure assessment. Additionally, there are important characteristics of laboratory tests (often referred to as "assays") that should be considered. For example, what is the lowest concentration that can be measured by the assay (often reported as the LOD, for limit of detection)? Is the expected range of concentrations able to be measured by the assay? How accurately does the assay measure known concentrations of the analyte? Most laboratory tests will report a coefficient of variation (CV) that assesses the variability of measured concentrations upon repeated testing of the same sample (calculated as mean/standard deviation and expressed as a percentage); the lower the CV, the closer the repeated measurements are to one another. You also should consider whether samples were measured in multiple batches (i.e., were samples all measured at a single point in time, or were they sent in smaller groups—"batches"—over a period of months or even years?). If the assays were performed on a series of batches, did the investigators consider potential variability across the batches? Finally, masking of laboratory personnel to outcome status is important in case-control studies.

How can I assess the accuracy of exposure assessment?

Sometimes exposure measurements can be highly valid, but oftentimes they have some level of error to them. Potential sources of error include biologic variation, inaccuracies in self-reporting (either intentional or unintentional), researcher errors in recording responses or measurements, computational errors, laboratory errors, or just random error.

Accuracy combines both the **reliability** of a measurement (i.e., does the measurement give the same answer every time) and the **validity** of the measurement (i.e., does the measurement actually measure what we are trying to measure). There are entire books written about assessing the validity and reliability of instruments, so it is not possible for us to cover all that here. Instead, let's talk about what to look for in an article to help you assess the accuracy of the exposure assessment.

One approach to assessing the validity of a test or instrument is to calculate its sensitivity and specificity compared to a gold standard. The higher the sensitivity, the lower the number of false negatives; the higher the specificity, the lower the number of false positives (refer to Chapter 2 for more information on how to calculate sensitivity and specificity). Ideally, we want the sensitivity and the specificity to be as close to 100% as possible.

Many established instruments have been "validated" against a gold standard, and authors will provide those details (or, at least cite a previous article reporting their results). For example, the Beck Depression Inventory (BDI) is a commonly used scale for assessing depression through a self-administered questionnaire. The BDI has been validated against structured clinical interviews, which are considered the gold standard for diagnosing clinical depression. These validation studies were used to establish the cut points of BDI scores that determine whether or not a patient has depression.[6]

Often, there is not an existing body of research on the validity of a measurement instrument. In this situation, the study authors might have conducted their own validation study on a subset of study subjects. For example, the investigators might have asked participants to self-report whether or not they have used antidepressant medications. Then, as an internal validation study, they could retrieve medical or pharmacy records on a randomly selected subset of participants (e.g., 10%) and check whether the self-reports match what is documented in the participants' records. Or, they might validate self-reported smoking status by measuring serum cotinine levels (a biomarker of cigarette smoking) in a random subsample of participants. If researchers can demonstrate high validity of the self-reports within the validation sub-study, then they would have confidence that the self-reported status in the full population is accurately reported as well.

Is the exposure that is measured the exposure that I care about?

Often, the exposure that needs to be measured is difficult, if not impossible, to measure directly. As a result, researchers develop ways to measure an exposure that gets them as close as possible to the desired exposure, while still being feasible for the study. In this sense, they are measuring a proxy of the potentially causal exposure.

When you consider exposure assessment in a study, your key concern is how closely the *measured* exposure reflects the *true* exposure the investigators seek to evaluate in relation to the outcome. You might consider the following questions to help you determine if the exposure that is measured represents the exposure that investigators were trying to measure:

- *Has the measurement approach been validated against a "gold standard" assessment for the exposure?* For example, a study validated self-reported tobacco use against serum cotinine measurements, which is considered the gold standard for measuring tobacco exposure.[7] Because their results showed high correspondence between the self-reports and the serum cotinine levels, the researchers demonstrated the validity of self-report for assessing regular tobacco use.
- *Does the measurement approach assess the actual exposure, or a marker of the actual exposure?* For example, a study seeking to evaluate the exposure of loneliness measured living alone as a marker for the actual exposure.[8] The survey analyzed for the study included questions about the participant's living situation but did not include any measurements of loneliness; researchers acknowledged that living alone does not necessarily mean someone is lonely (and, living with others does not necessarily mean someone is *not* lonely).
- *Does the measurement approach provide an assessment of the exposure at an appropriate time period?* For example, a prospective study of depression and antidepressant use in relation to breast cancer risk assessed current and previous

depression and antidepressant use at baseline and also repeatedly updated the status of these exposures throughout follow-up.[9] Updating exposure status was important because depression and antidepressant use are likely to change over time.

- *Are there important aspects of the exposure (e.g., timing, duration, dose) that need to be considered as part of the measurement approach?* For example, a prospective study evaluating perfluoroalkyl substances (PFAS) in relation to behavioral problems in children measured serum PFAS concentrations from maternal blood samples during pregnancy as well as in children's blood at ages 5 and 7 years.[10] Measuring PFAS exposure at multiple times allowed investigators to study the effects of PFAS exposure at different developmental stages.

What is misclassification?

Misclassification might sound confusing, but all it really means is that there is an error in the measurement. This error results in participants being placed into groups that don't reflect their true experiences.

Epidemiologic studies often seek to put participants into one of two groups: exposed or unexposed. Misclassification of exposure, then, means that the measurement approach causes some participants who are truly exposed to be erroneously put into the unexposed group, or vice versa. This can also happen in situations where the exposure is not just a question of "yes versus no" or "ever versus never." Many studies extend their classification of exposure to create more than two groups. For example, research exploring body mass index (BMI) as an exposure typically will classify participants into four groups: underweight (BMI <18.5 kg/m^2), normal weight (BMI $18.5–<25$ kg/m^2), overweight (BMI $25–<30$ kg/m^2), or obese (≥30 kg/m^2). In a situation like this, misclassification would mean that a participant is assigned to a different category by the measurement than is actually true. In other words, if someone who truly has a BMI $= 35.0$ kg/m^2 self-reports that their BMI is 25.0 kg/m^2, they would be misclassified as "overweight" when they really belong in the "obese" group.

Misclassification is a problem that weakens the internal validity of the study. But, the impact it has on the study's internal validity is determined by two things: (1) the extent to which misclassification occurs and (2) whether the misclassification is non-differential or differential. The first point likely makes intuitive sense: the more error (or misclassification) there is in a measurement, the more it will affect the study's results. The second point is harder to get your head wrapped around and will take some additional discussion. Briefly, the impact of exposure misclassification will depend on whether it is the same or different based on the participants' outcome status.

In this chapter, we will talk about misclassification of the exposure, but we will use the same terms to discuss misclassification in the outcome assessment in Chapter 7. Figure 6.1 shows a decision tree you can use to help you identify whether misclassification of exposure is present, and, if so, whether that misclassification is non-differential or differential.

What is non-differential misclassification of exposure?

Simply put, **non-differential misclassification of exposure** is when the error in the exposure measurement equally affects both those with and those without the outcome. In other words, there is "no difference" in the likelihood (or probability) of

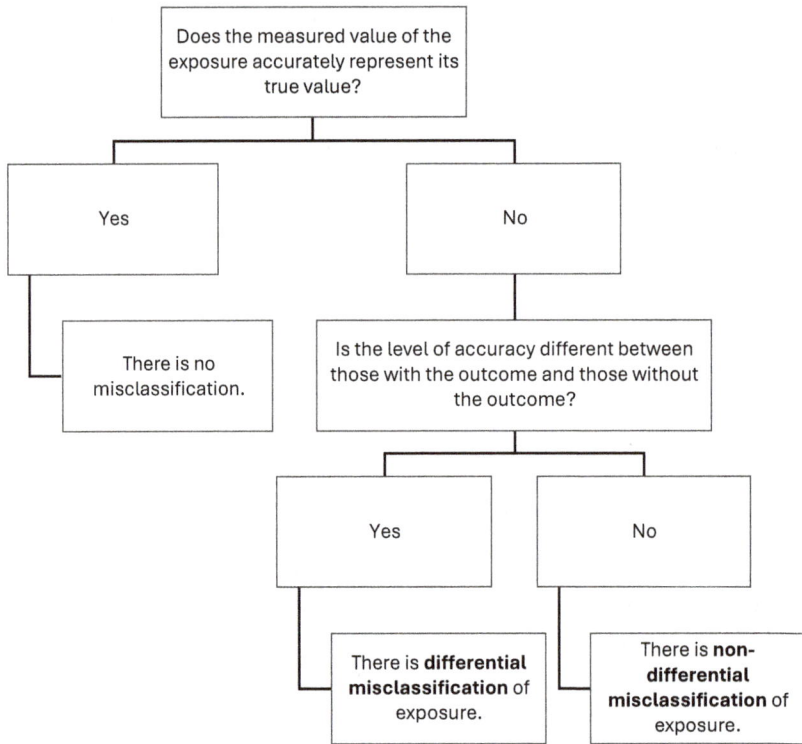

Figure 6.1 Exposure misclassification occurs whenever the measured value of an exposure is not equal to its true value. Differential and non-differential misclassification have important implications for the internal validity of a study. This decision-tree can be helpful for distinguishing between differential and non-differential misclassification.

misclassification between cases and controls (in a case-control study) or between those who eventually develop or do not develop the outcome (in prospective study designs).

As an example, imagine that you are running a case-control study in which you want to evaluate whether body weight is associated with the outcome. For the moment, let's set aside the (very appropriate) criticism that measuring body weight after diagnosis would not be causally related to the development of the outcome, and instead focus on how weight would be measured. Imagine an extreme example in which you have two research nurses who use different scales to measure the participants' weight (Figure 6.2). If everyone has their weight measured with a perfectly calibrated scale, there would be no exposure misclassification from this measurement approach. However, if one scale is perfectly calibrated, while the other is not and adds anywhere between 5 and 10 pounds to each person's weight, you would have exposure misclassification. If the nurse and the scale that measures a participant's weight have nothing to do with whether they are a case or a control, then cases and controls are equally likely to have their weight misclassified. Because there is no difference in the probability of misclassification of weight between the cases and controls, you would say that there is non-differential misclassification of exposure.

Generally speaking, epidemiologists worry a lot less about non-differential misclassification than we do about its counterpart, differential misclassification. A big part of

A. All cases and all controls have weight measured with a perfectly calibrated scale

No misclassification of exposure

B. Some cases and some controls have their weight measured with a perfectly calibrated scale, while the rest have their weight measured with an uncalibrated scale that adds 5-10 lbs.

Non-differential misclassification of exposure

C. All cases have their weight measured with a perfectly calibrated scale, while all controls have their weight measured with an uncalibrated scale that adds 5-10 lbs.

Differential misclassification of exposure

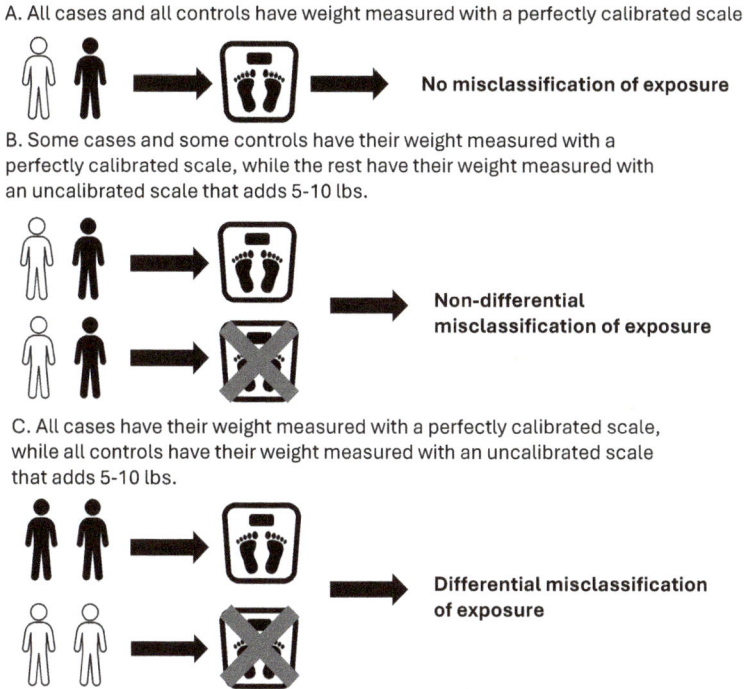

Figure 6.2 Exposure misclassification occurs when there is a difference between the exposure's true value and its measured value. Consider an extreme example, in which a case-control study exploring body weight as the exposure measures weight in a clinic. If weight is measured for all participants using a perfectly calibrated scale, there would be no misclassification due to the scale (A). However, if some participants have their weight measured with an uncalibrated scale, and there is no relationship between case/control status and which scale is used, then there would be non-differential misclassification of exposure (B). Finally, if all the cases have their weight measured with the perfectly calibrated scale, while all the controls have their weight measured using the uncalibrated scale, there would be differential misclassification of exposure (C).

the reason is that non-differential misclassification tends to make the groups appear to be more similar than they really are, and this tends to skew our results toward the null hypothesis (i.e., no difference). While this is nearly always true when exposure is classified as exposed or unexposed, it is not always the case when exposure is classified into more than two categories. But, as a rule of thumb, we can anticipate that in most situations, non-differential misclassification will tend to skew results toward the null hypothesis. In other words, any observed association might actually be weaker than what would have been observed if there had not been non-differential misclassification of the exposure.

What is differential misclassification of exposure?

Now that we know that non-differential misclassification means that there is no difference in the accuracy of exposure assessment between those with and those without the outcome, it shouldn't be surprising that **differential misclassification of exposure** means that there is a difference in the accuracy of exposure assessment between those with and those without the outcome. You might have been taught the terms **information bias** or **observation bias**; these are essentially synonyms for differential misclassification. Returning to the previous example of the two scales, differential misclassification of exposure would occur if all the cases had their weight measured with the perfectly calibrated scale, while all the controls had their weight measured with the uncalibrated scale (Panel C in Figure 6.2). Admittedly, this is an extreme example, and one that you are unlikely to encounter in a published journal article. Most instances of differential misclassification of exposure are less obvious (but, thinking through extreme examples can be helpful for understanding the concept itself).

Differential misclassification of exposure is far more worrisome than non-differential misclassification of exposure. Because the level of misclassification differs between those with and without the outcome (or, those with different levels of risk of the outcome), the direction of effect on the estimated association is harder to predict. Differential misclassification of exposure can skew results either toward the null hypothesis or away from the null hypothesis. Because it has the potential to make it appear that there is an association when there truly is not an association, differential misclassification of exposure is a particularly serious threat to internal validity.

As an example, consider a case-control study that explored associations between genital talc use and ovarian cancer.[11] Scientists had been investigating a potential link between talc and ovarian cancer since at least the 1990s, but with inconclusive results. This particular case-control study recruited women diagnosed with ovarian cancer from 2010 to 2015; however, in 2014 multiple class action lawsuits were filed against the company that manufactured talcum powder. As a result, public awareness of the idea that talc might cause ovarian cancer rose sharply. Investigators were concerned that cases might over-report talc exposure due to their awareness of the lawsuits. To assess this potential recall bias (i.e., differential misclassification), they stratified their analysis based on whether participants were interviewed before or after 2014. The results were quite striking. Among participants interviewed before 2014, there was no statistically significant association between any genital talc use and ovarian cancer (OR 1.19, 95% CI 0.87–1.63). However, among participants interviewed *after* 2014, there was nearly a threefold increase in risk (OR 2.91, 95% CI 1.70–4.97). You can reasonably conclude that the participants diagnosed with ovarian cancer and interviewed after 2014 likely over-reported their prior genital talc use given the widespread media attention on the lawsuits. Recall bias in action!

How does exposure misclassification happen in studies?

It would be impossible to identify every possible circumstance in which exposure misclassification could occur. But, there are some common situations that you can recognize as being susceptible to exposure misclassification:

- The exposure is measured at a time that is not relevant to disease development (e.g., measuring serum cholesterol *after* diagnosis in a case-control study).
- The exposure status changes over time, yet is only assessed once (e.g., measuring BMI at enrollment in a prospective cohort study with 20 years of follow-up).
- The outcome under study is known to have a critical window of susceptibility, yet the exposure measurement isn't measured during that time period (e.g., pregnancy

is a critical window of susceptibility for neural tube defects in infants, thus measuring exposures after birth would be irrelevant).

- The disease itself and/or the process of being diagnosed and treated for the disease affects the exposure status (e.g., sleep, physical activity, and diet all often change prior to cancer diagnosis and continue to be affected by diagnosis and treatment).
- The exposure assessment is via self-report, but the exposure is difficult to recall accurately. This is especially problematic in case-control studies, where recall bias can occur because cases tend to remember and/or report differently (either more accurately or less accurately) than controls (e.g., ovarian cancer cases recall talcum powder use differently than controls due to awareness of potential links following class action lawsuits).
- The exposure is stigmatized, such that participants might be unwilling to report honestly (e.g., illicit drug use, sexual history).
- The study uses different measurement approaches based on outcome status (e.g., proxy reports for cases vs self-report for controls).
- The definition of exposure is too broad (e.g., smoking is classified as "ever" vs "never", which means that there is a wide range of smoking exposure among the "ever" group).

When I read an article, how do I evaluate exposure misclassification?

As you read an epidemiologic article, you will want to pay close attention to how the exposure is measured. This should be described thoroughly in the Methods section, and many articles will create a subsection specifically for describing the exposure assessment. Thinking through the following questions will likely help you identify the strengths and limitations of the exposure assessment and evaluate their impact on internal validity:

- *Does the measurement represent the (potentially) causal exposure, or is it a proxy or marker of that exposure?*
- *Has the exposure measurement been validated against a gold standard?*
- *Is the exposure measurement reliable?*
- *If the exposure is categorized into multiple groups, is the range of exposure within each group too broad or too narrow?*
- *Does the exposure measurement reflect the etiologically relevant time period?*
- *Was exposure measured before or after outcome status was determined?*
- *Were the same methods used to assess exposure in cases and controls (in case-control studies) or in various subgroups that may have a different risk of disease (in prospective cohort studies)?*
- *Could the outcome under study have affected the biological levels being measured?*
- *Could the outcome under study, especially pre-symptomatic disease, have affected the exposure?*

Additionally, examining the results presented in the article can often provide important information for assessing the potential for error and bias in the exposure measurement. As you read through the Results section and examine the Tables, considering the following questions can be helpful:

■ *Do the reported associations between the exposure and other factors (e.g., age, education, other outcomes) match what you would expect based on prior studies?*

■ *Does the study provide results of analyses intended to examine the impact of potential sources of bias (e.g., repeating analyses excluding proxy-reported exposures), and, if so, are the results of these analyses similar to those of the primary analyses?*

■ *How do results change when different measures of the exposure are used (e.g., self-report vs medical records) or when different classifications of the exposure are used (e.g., including as a continuous variable vs categorizing into groups reflecting different exposure ranges)?*

■ *For randomized controlled trials, was adherence to assigned treatment group reported, and was it high?*

STAR in action: examining the exposure in Mirick et al.

Table 6.2 shows how the STAR template can be used to critically evaluate the exposure assessment used in the Mirick et al.[12] article. The primary exposure is regular use of antiperspirants or deodorants. Participants provided this information through an in-person interview.

There is some potential for recall bias, as cases might have different recalls of these exposures if they are aware that antiperspirants/deodorants are hypothesized to increase breast cancer risk. It is not known whether interviewers were masked to case/control status, so interviewer bias is possible. Overall, there is a moderate possibility of differential misclassification due to recall bias and/or interviewer bias.

Additionally, there is a moderate to major concern for non-differential misclassification of exposure. All participants may have difficulty recalling their lifetime use of these products, especially older participants. Furthermore, only participants who

Table 6.2 Completed STAR template Section 3: "Exposure Assessment" for Mirick et al. (2002)[12]

Exposure assessment	
Describe (i.e., report just the facts described in the article)	Critique (i.e., think through strengths/limitations of the methods and results; address the key questions listed, and add additional comments as needed)
What was the primary exposure of interest?	Is this exposure appropriate for addressing the stated objective?
Regular use of antiperspirant or deodorant	**Yes, exposure matches that in the stated exposure**
Also assessed if these products were used regularly within 1 hour of underarm shaving	

(Continued)

Table 6.2 (*Continued*)

Exposure assessment

How was the primary exposure measured? Be specific—include details of measurement tools, assays, and used.	Was the measurement of exposure reliable? Was the measurement of exposure valid? What strengths and/or limitations do you note?
	Exposure assessment based on self-report, with no possible way to validate; however, exposure is fairly straightforward and likely something that participants could understand and report accurately, especially for ever/never using these products
In-person interview; participants who responded that they routinely shaved their underarms were asked further questions about antiperspirant use, deodorant use, talc product use, and if products were applied within 1 hour of shaving	Strengths: in-person interviews reduce missing data, standard questionnaire used for cases and controls
	Limitation: possible social desirability bias (participants may answer based on what is culturally "normal" rather than what is true for them)
	Could the study results have been affected by **differential** misclassification of exposure? Why or why not? If so, describe direction, magnitude, and likelihood.
	Moderate potential for recall bias causing differential misclassification; breast cancer cases may be more likely to remember their previous deodorant/antiperspirant usage and duration compared to the controls because they might be more aware of possible risk factors of breast cancer and searching for a reason for their cancer diagnosis; would likely bias away from the null hypothesis
	Also, possible that interview bias could cause differential misclassification; no mention of masking to disease status, so possible that interview may have probed more (or less) for cases vs controls, especially if interviewers were aware of study hypothesis; could bias toward or away from null depending on particular situation and which group is over-/under-reporting
	Could the study results have been affected by **nondifferential** misclassification of the exposure? Why or why not? If so, describe direction, magnitude and likelihood.
	Yes, would occur if cases and controls are equally likely to report their antiperspirant/deodorant use inaccurately (either over- or under-reporting)
	Since participants were asked to recall their exposure from their past "lifetime," which for older participants might be difficult to remember accurately.
	Also, deodorant/antiperspirant questions were only asked if participants reporting shaved underarms; anyone who did not shave therefore either had missing data and was not included or was classified as "no" for deodorant/antiperspirant use; 94% of cases and 93% of controls reported underarm shaving, however, making this a minor concern

(*Continued*)

Table 6.2 (*Continued*)

Exposure assessment
Overall, non-differential misclassification would have a minor/moderate impact for a simpler classification like ever/never regular use, and a moderate/major impact for a harder-to-remember exposure like use within 1 hour of shaving, on the study's finding, tending to bias toward the null
Note any additional comments: none

responded that they regularly shaved their underarms were asked about antiperspirant and deodorant use. The article does not clearly state whether participants who did not shave were excluded from the analysis or if they were classified as "no"; if the latter, then there is a possibility of non-differential misclassification. However, because 94% of cases and 93% of controls reported underarm shaving, this is only a minor concern. Importantly, there is a lack of specific information on frequency and duration of product use and also categorizing essentially as ever versus never, which lacks information on use during specific periods of susceptibility that are relevant to future breast cancer risk. It is also possible that participants reported their current use of these products, which may not reflect their use prior to breast cancer diagnosis or a similar historical period for controls. Overall, non-differential misclassification of exposure could have a moderate/major impact on the study's finding, tending to bias toward the null.

Activities
Find a recently published observational study or randomized controlled trial on a topic of interest to you. You might consider using the article you read for the Activities from Chapter 5.

1. Complete Section 3 of the STAR template for this article to describe how the exposure was measured and evaluate the potential for bias and error.
2. Based on your answers to the questions in the STAR template, evaluate how the exposure assessment affects the internal validity of the study.
3. Think about other approaches to exposure assessment for the exposure of interest in the article. How might these other approaches serve to either strengthen or limit internal validity? Would these approaches be more or less feasible, given the study design and study population under study in the article?

References
1. Brazier JE, Harper R, Jones NM, et al. Validating the SF-36 health survey questionnaire: New outcome measure for primary care. *BMJ*. 1992;305(6846):160–164.
2. Anderson C, Laubscher S, Burns R. Validation of the short form 36 (SF-36) health survey questionnaire among stroke patients. *Stroke*. 1996;27(10):1812–1816. doi:10.1161/01. STR.27.10.1812
3. Lyons RA, Perry HM, Littlepage BN. Evidence for the validity of the short-form 36 questionnaire (SF-36) in an elderly population. *Age Ageing*. 1994;23(3):182–184. doi:10.1093/ageing/23.3.182

4. Coons S, Al Abdulmohsin SA, Draugalis JR, Hays RD. Reliability of an Arabic version of the RAND-36 health survey and its equivalence to the US-English version. *Med Care.* Published online January 1, 1998. Accessed July 22, 2024. https://www.rand.org/pubs/external_publications/EP19980309.html

5. Arocho R, McMillan CA. Discriminant and criterion validation of the US-Spanish version of the SF-36 Health Survey in a Cuban-American population with benign prostatic hyperplasia. *Med Care.* 1998;36(5):766–772. doi:10.1097/00005650–199805000-00017

6. Kendall PC, Hollon SD, Beck AT, Hammen CL, Ingram RE. Issues and recommendations regarding use of the Beck Depression Inventory. *Cogn Ther Res.* 1987;11(3):289–299. doi:10.1007/BF01186280

7. Zettergren A, Sompa S, Palmberg L, et al. Assessing tobacco use in Swedish young adults from self-report and urinary cotinine: A validation study using the BAMSE birth cohort. *BMJ Open.* 2023;13(7):e072582. doi:10.1136/bmjopen-2023–072582

8. Olfson M, Cosgrove CM, Altekruse SF, Wall MM, Blanco C. Living alone and suicide risk in the United States, 2008–2019. *Am J Public Health.* 2022;112(12):1774–1782. doi:10.2105/AJPH.2022.307080

9. Reeves KW, Okereke OI, Qian J, Tamimi RM, Eliassen AH, Hankinson SE. Depression, antidepressant use, and breast cancer risk in pre- and postmenopausal women: A prospective cohort study. *Cancer Epidemiol Biomarkers Prev.* 2018;27(3):306–314. doi:10.1158/1055–9965.EPI-17-0707

10. Oulhote Y, Steuerwald U, Debes F, Weihe P, Grandjean P. Behavioral difficulties in 7-year old children in relation to developmental exposure to perfluorinated alkyl substances. *Environ Int.* 2016;97:237–245. doi:10.1016/j.envint.2016.09.015

11. Schildkraut JM, Abbott SE, Alberg AJ, et al. Association between body powder use and ovarian cancer: The African American Cancer Epidemiology study (AACES). *Cancer Epidemiol Biomark Prev.* 2016;25(10):1411–1417. doi:10.1158/1055–9965.EPI-15–1281

12. Mirick DK, Davis S, Thomas DB. Antiperspirant use and the risk of breast cancer. *J Natl Cancer Inst.* 2002;94(20):1578–1580. doi:10.1093/jnci/94.20.1578

CHAPTER 7

How was the outcome measured?

In many epidemiologic studies, the outcome being studied is a specific disease. Either the person has the disease, or they do not. You might think that disease is pretty easy to measure and that this will be a short chapter. Unfortunately, you'd be wrong on both accounts.

In reality, determining who does and does not have the outcome under study can be complicated. Some diseases and conditions require specialized (and potentially expensive) testing for diagnosis, which may not be readily available to all segments of the population (e.g., individuals without health insurance may not be able to access colon cancer screening tests, including colonoscopies). Other diseases and conditions may be asymptomatic, meaning that many people who think they are unaffected might actually have the disease (e.g., COVID-19, especially early in the pandemic prior to the widespread availability of testing). Still, other diseases have many sub-types and can be confusing for non-medical professionals to understand and accurately report which one they have (e.g., some people with benign breast disease will misreport their diagnosis as breast cancer). And, sometimes the way we measure the outcome impacts whether we are counting all cases of disease or only the most severe (e.g., defining "asthma" based only on emergency room visits would miss out on less severe cases of asthma, which do not result in a trip to the hospital).

If you want to draw accurate conclusions from a study's results, it is important to fully understand how the investigators defined and measured the outcome. Similar to what we discussed with measuring the exposure, there is often more than one approach that could be used to measure the outcome. Imagine that your research team wanted to conduct a study to evaluate risk factors for depression (Table 7.1). You might consider measuring depression by: (1) having participants self-report feelings of depression within the past 4 weeks, (2) asking participants to self-report a clinical diagnosis of depression, (3) measuring depressive symptoms using a validated scale (e.g., the Beck Depression Inventory), or (4) reviewing primary care provider records for a diagnosis of depression. Your research team would need to carefully consider the strengths and

DOI: 10.4324/9781003637899-8

Table 7.1 There often are multiple approaches that could be used to measure a given outcome. For example, "depression" could be measured through self-report of feeling depressed or of a clinical diagnosis, through administering a validated scale to measure depressive symptoms, or through primary care provider records. Each approach has both strengths and limitations, and investigators weigh these as they select a measurement approach for their study

Approach for measuring depression	Strengths	Limitations
Self-reported feelings of depression within past 4 weeks *Self- or interviewer-administered questionnaire, asking about feelings of depression in prior 4 weeks*	■ Measuring "current" depressive symptoms ■ Easy, fast, and not expensive	■ Depressive symptoms are different from a clinical diagnosis of depression ■ Only measures depression within prior 4 weeks ■ Cases that have resolved will be missed if only asking once ■ Unable to distinguish severity or duration of depression ■ Neither sensitivity nor specificity would be very high ■ Prone to social desirability bias
Self-reported clinical diagnosis of depression *Self- or interviewer-administered questionnaire, asking "have you ever been diagnosed with depression by a health care provider"*	■ Measures cases that result in a clinical diagnosis ■ May also be able to inquire about dates of diagnosis to assess duration ■ Easy, fast, and not expensive	■ Participants' access to care will affect ascertainment ■ Participants' willingness to seek care will affect ascertainment ■ Prone to social desirability bias
Measure depressive symptoms using a validated scale *Administer a questionnaire such as Beck Depression Inventory*	■ Scale has been validated against a gold standard clinical interview ■ Facilitates comparison with other studies that have used the same scale for measuring depression ■ Easy, fast, and not expensive	■ Depressive symptoms are not equivalent to a clinical diagnosis of depression ■ Participants who have clinical depression and are being effectively treated won't score as depressed on the scale, thus cases would be misclassified ■ Cases that have resolved will be missed ■ Only measures current depressive symptoms ■ Unable to distinguish duration of depression
Review primary care provider records for depression diagnosis *Access participants' medical records and look for ICD codes appropriate for depression diagnoses*	■ Definitive in terms of significant clinical depression ■ Ensures consistency across participants because of ICD codes	■ Participant access to care will affect ascertainment ■ Participant willingness to seek care will affect ascertainment ■ Requires significant resources to review medical records

limitations of these approaches, and then select the one that is both most valid and most feasible for your study.

Ideally, studies would be 100% accurate in measuring their specified outcome, and there would be no differences in the accuracy of this measurement by exposure status and/or other important characteristics of the source and/or study population. But by now you know that epidemiologic studies are never perfect. There is always an opportunity for bias and error when you are measuring humans.

In this chapter, we will take a deep dive into outcome ascertainment, with a focus on opportunities for bias and error to sneak in and distort results. The concepts presented here are equally applicable across all study designs. In other words, considering how the outcome was measured is just as important in a case-control study as it is for a randomized controlled trial.

What do epidemiologists mean by "outcome" anyway?

Even though it is one of the key pieces of an epidemiologic study, the term outcome can be confusing to students. Often when I ask students to identify the outcome of the study, they respond by citing odds ratios and the study's main conclusions. Although it makes sense that they would interpret the word "outcome" to mean the results reported in the study, "outcome" has a very precise—and very different—meaning in epidemiology. Because the outcome of a study could be any number of factors, students often have trouble identifying the outcome when reading a manuscript.

Back in Chapter 2, I defined **outcome** as the disease or condition under study. For example, an outcome could be the diagnosis of Alzheimer's disease. Or, the outcome could be a condition such as osteoporosis, identified based on one's bone mineral density. Sometimes, though, the outcome can be something other than a disease or condition. For example, you may want to study predictors of adherence to a new medication or treatment. In that case, the outcome would not be the disease or condition that is being treated but rather would be adherence (i.e., whether or not the patients take their medication or treatment as prescribed).

How was the outcome measured in the study?

There are many common approaches to measuring the outcome. Some of these include: (1) self-report, (2) administering a diagnostic questionnaire or diagnostic test, (3) reviewing medical records, and (4) using external registries and reporting databases. Sometimes, investigators will use a combination of these approaches as a way of assessing the outcome (e.g., defining hypertension as measured high blood pressure in the clinic or documented high blood pressure in the participant's medical record). Let's consider each one of these approaches in turn, paying careful attention to their strengths and limitations.

Self-report

Most of the time, the easiest way to determine if someone has a specific outcome is to just ask them. This works very well for some outcomes, and less well for others. Outcomes that most people can report accurately are often ones that are straightforward to diagnose and are life-changing enough that people know and understand their diagnosis. For example, if the outcome in a study of pregnant women is "full-term live birth," the study participants very likely can report if they had a full-term live birth or not with a high degree of accuracy.

But, even seemingly easily self-reported conditions sometimes can become problematic. For example, if we ask participants "have you ever been told by a health care professional that you have melanoma (an invasive form of skin cancer)?" some people who have a history of benign (i.e., non-melanoma) skin cancers will answer "yes." It is fairly common for people to misunderstand the difference between melanoma and benign skin cancers; they might just remember that their dermatologist told them they had a cancerous lesion that needed to be removed. Likewise, someone who had pre-cancerous colorectal polyps removed during a colonoscopy might inaccurately report that they had colorectal cancer.

For outcomes in which a substantial proportion of affected people are asymptomatic, including disease that is asymptomatic in only early stages and/or disease that remains asymptomatic for some people, this too can cause inaccuracy in self-reported outcome assessments. For example, hypertension is often asymptomatic, and cases may be unaware that they have hypertension unless they have their blood pressure checked.

Administering a diagnostic questionnaire or diagnostic test

Many studies will measure the outcome by administering their own assessment. This might consist of asking participants to complete a questionnaire that includes a validated scale for measuring the outcome (e.g., the Beck Depression Inventory to measure depression), or it might mean performing a clinical assessment (e.g., measuring blood pressure to evaluate presence or absence of hypertension).

There are important benefits to this approach for the outcome assessment. First, it does not rely on the participant's memory or understanding of their diagnosis. Second, investigators can ensure that everyone is given the same test and thus reduce the chances of non-differential misclassification of outcome (more on what that means soon). Third, if the assessment has been independently validated, this gives reassurance that the outcome is being measured accurately (more on validation and sensitivity/ specificity soon too).

As with any approach, though, there are some limitations. First, even a validated assessment can have errors. Unless both sensitivity and specificity of the instrument are 100%, some people will be misclassified.

Second, for some diseases and conditions, effective treatment will reduce or eliminate symptoms. If these symptoms are measured by the instrument to identify presence of the condition, then the instrument will not recognize that the participant has the disease or condition under study. For example, someone who is effectively treated for depression with antidepressants or therapy likely will not report depressive symptoms on the Beck Depression Inventory. Likewise, someone effectively treated for hypertension with anti-hypertensive agents will not have elevated blood pressure when measured in the clinic. In both examples, the effective treatment masks the presence of the condition, and individuals with depression or hypertension would be classified as *not* having those outcomes.

Third, for conditions where patients recover and potentially relapse, a test given at one moment in time may not capture the outcome accurately. For example, a patient with depression as a teenager may no longer experience depression in adulthood. Depending on whether you are looking to measure whether a participant "currently" has the outcome or has "ever" had the outcome, a depression assessment of that participant as an adult could misclassify them. In other words, if you are interested in studying "ever had depression" as your outcome, measuring depression with the Beck Depression Inventory at one point in time as an adult would not capture the prior experiences with depression as a teenager.

Fourth, the resources (of time, money, equipment, and/or personnel) needed to administer the diagnostic questionnaire or test may not be available, making this approach infeasible. Lastly, if the diagnostic test requires participants to provide a blood sample or to have a specialized medical examination, this increases the burden placed on the participant. Some individuals, in fact, may be less inclined to participate if they know that doing so means having blood drawn or an x-ray performed.

Reviewing medical records or other existing records

Medical records could include records from a primary care physician, hospital records, pharmacy records, health insurance records, or any other documentation related to receipt of medical care. Generally speaking, medical records are an excellent approach for gathering information about the outcome. If it is documented in the medical record, you can have a high degree of confidence that the participant truly has the disease or condition. Sometimes investigators can even access specific test results (e.g., pathology reports, radiology reports) to verify the diagnosis for themselves. Additionally, the use of standard International Classification of Diseases (ICD) codes can further ensure that outcomes are captured correctly and consistently.

Although the strengths of medical records are impressive, there are some limitations to consider as well. While some countries have universal healthcare and excellent databases that can be used to identify outcomes, not all do. In particular, access to medical care in the U.S. varies greatly across groups defined by many characteristics, including race/ethnicity, gender, health insurance status, and geographic location. Even if it is possible to access medical care, access to highly specialized care needed to accurately diagnose certain conditions could still be limited. Additionally, it may be challenging to access medical records if participants are not all recruited from the same clinic, hospital, or health insurance company. Some participants may not consent to allowing investigators to access their medical records, which would lead to missing data. Furthermore, the U.S. healthcare system is not a single network, meaning that diagnoses made by one provider at a certain medical facility may not necessarily be recorded in the health records at a patient's other health care providers who provide care at other facilities. Such discrepancies could be a result of electronic health records systems not communicating with one another, or could also arise if patients are selective about discussing certain conditions with various health care providers (e.g., a patient who opts not to disclose their depression, diagnosed by a primary care provider, with the specialist they see once a year).

External registries and databases

Many diseases are recorded through external registries and databases. You'll recall from Chapter 4 that disease surveillance is important for monitoring public health trends. Oftentimes we can use these same resources to measure outcomes on participants. For example, some case-control studies might recruit cases from cancer registries. An additional advantage of outcome ascertainment from disease registries is that they often have a great deal of information about the case, including date of diagnosis and biological characteristics of the disease (e.g., stage, grade, prognostic molecular, and/or genetic features). Also, registries for diseases with mandated reporting often have excellent coverage over a defined area (e.g., state, county). When controls are recruited from the geographic area covered by the registry, you can feel confident that they pass the "would" test. In other words, it is very likely that if these individuals were diagnosed with the disease, they "would" have been identified as a case (note: this is not a question of outcome misclassification, but rather a reassurance against selection bias).

However, not all external records and registries are equally accurate. Issues with data from death certificates, which are generally available through government records, are well documented.[1] For example, consider someone who dies in a car crash that occurred following their fatal stroke while driving. Unless an autopsy is performed, their cause of death might be recorded as trauma due to the car crash, when the true cause of death was the stroke.

What does it mean for the outcome to have misclassification?

Remember that misclassification is any situation where the measured (i.e., observed) value is different than the true value. When we talk about **outcome misclassification**, we mean that someone who has the outcome is classified as not having the outcome, or vice versa; this could be a result of errors in diagnosis or could be a result of errors in reporting. As we have seen from the above discussion of strengths and limitations of various approaches to outcome assessment, misclassification of outcomes can arise through a variety of factors. Having a clear, specific, and consistently applied definition of the outcome under study can help to reduce misclassification.

As you might expect, outcome misclassification can have an important impact on the internal validity of the study's findings. The extent to which outcome misclassification affects the study results will depend on two things: (1) the level of misclassification that has occurred, and (2) if the misclassification was differential or non-differential in nature. Let's take a closer look at each of these issues in turn. Similar to exposure misclassification, you can use a decision-tree to help you determine if there is outcome misclassification (Figure 7.1).

How can I assess the accuracy of outcome assessment?

Common sense tells us that if 50% of your outcomes are misclassified, you have a problem; this should definitely be put into your "major issue" bucket. But, if only if 0.1% of your outcomes are misclassified, then you could rightly put this into your "minor issue" bucket. So, how do you figure out what the extent of outcome misclassification is in the study?

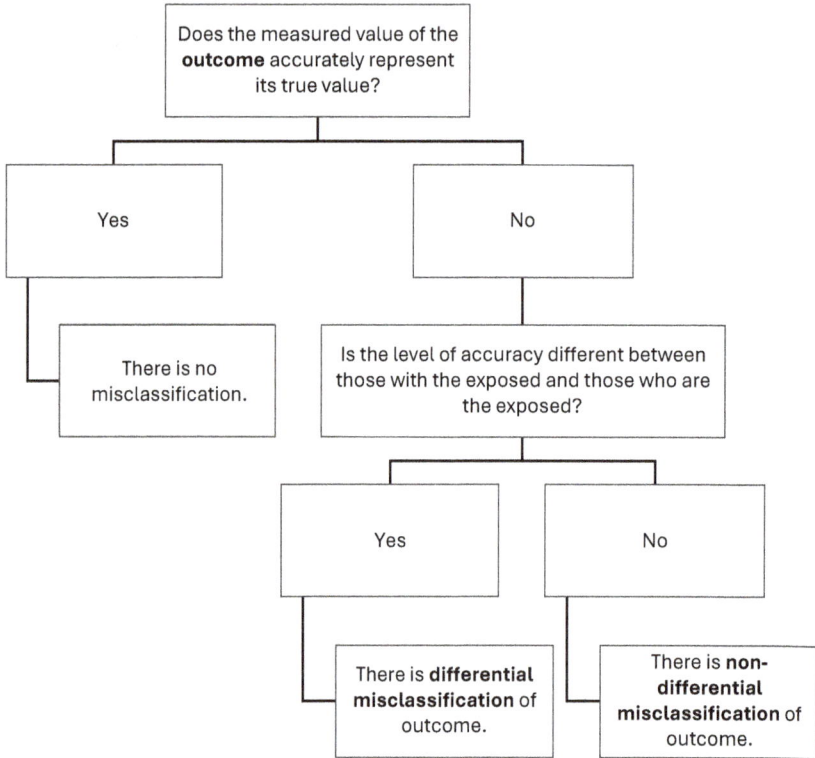

Figure 7.1 Outcome misclassification occurs whenever the measured value of an outcome is not equal to its true value. For example, a participant with the outcome is measured to not have the outcome. Differential and non-differential misclassification have important implications for the internal validity of a study. This decision-tree can be helpful for distinguishing between differential and non-differential misclassification of outcomes.

Recall that in Chapter 6 we talked about the accuracy of measurement approach as a combination of its validity (i.e., does the measurement measure what we are trying to measure?) and its reliability (i.e., does the measurement give the same answer every time?). Much of the time, outcomes are assessed using a set of standard diagnostic criteria and/or identified through ICD codes. These approaches can be regarded as highly accurate, although to some extent they do rely on the expertise of the medical professional to correctly diagnose the condition.

Often, diseases and conditions are identified through screening tests, for example, a mammogram to detect breast cancer. The sensitivity and specificity of screening tests are well-established before the tests are widely adopted. If the authors of the article don't cite the test's sensitivity and specificity, you can easily find them yourself through a literature search on PubMed,[2] referring to evaluations made by the U.S. Preventive Services Task Force,[3] or using other tools available to medical and health professionals (e.g., Cochrane Reviews[4] and UpToDate[5]).

Not all approaches to assessing outcomes have been extensively validated, however. As we discussed with exposure assessment, small validation studies are often conducted within a study to evaluate the validity of the approach to outcome assessment. For example, the Study of Women's Health Across the Nation followed 3,302 women beginning in 1996. Approximately once per year, participants self-reported newly diagnosed cases of breast cancer. As noted earlier, self-report is generally a less valid approach to outcome assessment than using medical records. Years after the study began, investigators studying breast cancer outcomes wanted to assess the validity of these self-reports. However, it was not possible for the study investigators to retrieve medical records on all participants. In a small validation study, though, the investigators retrieved medical records (including pathology reports and radiology reports) on a subset of 80 women who had self-reported a breast cancer diagnosis. The validation study showed that 95% of self-reported breast cancer cases were accurately reported, which led them to conclude that the self-reported breast cancer cases had minimal outcome misclassification.[6]

What is non-differential misclassification of outcome?

Similar to what we discussed with exposure misclassification, "non-differential" means the level of misclassification is *equivalent* between groups. With outcome misclassification, the groups are defined by exposure status. So, **non-differential misclassification of outcome** means that the extent of misclassification among the exposed and the unexposed groups is equal.

For example, the sensitivity of chest x-rays as a screening tool for lung cancer is approximately 75%,[7] meaning that roughly 25% of true lung cancer cases will be misclassified as non-cases (i.e., false negatives) on a screening chest x-ray. If everyone in the study, without any regard for their exposure status, is given a chest x-ray to screen for lung cancer, then the resulting outcome misclassification would be non-differential. This is shown in panel A of Figure 7.2: both smokers and non-smokers with lung cancer are given a chest x-ray, and one out of every four cases in each group is missed by this test. The misclassification is similar for smokers and non-smokers, so the misclassification is non-differential. Non-differential misclassification of outcome tends to bias estimated associations toward the null.

What is differential misclassification of outcome?

Differential misclassification of outcome occurs when the level of misclassification is *different* between groups. As we noted above, when we consider the outcome, the groups are defined by the exposure status. It could be that the outcome is classified more accurately among the exposed, or it could be the opposite.

As an example, let's return to our scenario of the chest x-ray to screen for lung cancer. We already have established that chest x-rays will miss about one in four lung cancer cases. In panel B of Figure 7.2, smokers are more likely to be offered lung cancer screening by their primary care providers than non-smokers due to their known high lung cancer risk from their smoking history. Imagine, then, if you have a group of individuals who all truly have lung cancer; some of these people are smokers, and some are non-smokers. You are more likely to misclassify the outcome status of the non-smokers because they were not given the screening test. So, if you are relying on routine medical care to identify lung cancer diagnoses in a prospective cohort study, you would be very likely to miss lung cancers that occur among non-smokers. At a minimum, new lung

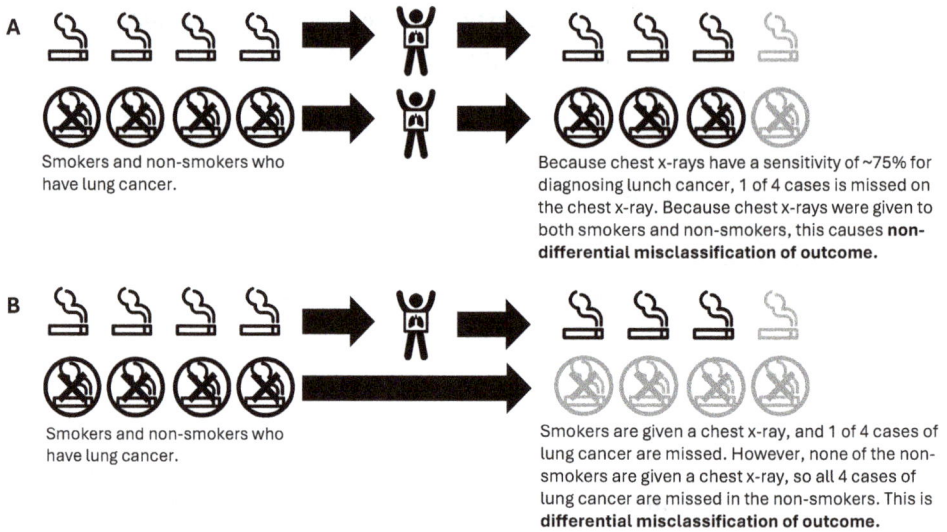

Figure 7.2 Chest x-rays as a screening test for lung cancer have ~75% sensitivity. As a result, some lung cancer cases will be misclassified as non-cases if outcome assessment is based on chest x-ray screening. If exposure (e.g., smoking status) is unrelated to who receives a chest x-ray, this will cause non-differential misclassification of exposure (A). However, if only smokers are given chest x-rays and non-smokers are not given chest x-rays, then there will be differential misclassification of outcome (B).

cancers found in non-smokers would be at a later stage, because of the lack of secondary screening to identify asymptomatic disease.

Differential misclassification of outcomes can bias estimates toward or away from the null hypothesis. To determine the direction of its effect on our estimated measure of association, we need to think through the scenario at hand and figure out whether the outcome is over-diagnosed or under-diagnosed in the different exposure groups. This can become rather complicated, so we will not tackle this topic here. Instead, I'll refer interested readers to excellent discussions found in intermediate and advanced epidemiology textbooks (e.g., *Modern Epidemiology*[8] and *Gordis Epidemiology*[9]).

How does outcome misclassification happen in studies?

To identify outcome misclassification, it is helpful to think through the entire process by which a participant would be identified as having the outcome, including how their decisions and/or behaviors (and those of others, including health care professionals) could affect whether or not they receive a diagnosis. Doing so helps you to identify possible sources of error (or, to identify procedures that reduce the likelihood of errors). Outcome misclassification can occur from any number of processes that have gone wrong. While it would be impossible to create an exhaustive list, you can identify some common reasons for outcome misclassification to occur:

■ *Clerical or laboratory errors*. For example, a positive test result gets inaccurately recorded in the medical record as a negative result. Or, the laboratory test is misread as negative when it is actually positive. It may be hard to believe, but these types of errors do occur.

■ *Sensitivity and specificity of the medical test or diagnostic criteria being used.* We saw earlier how chest x-rays will miss about one in four lung cancer cases due to their 75% sensitivity. Unless a screening test or diagnostic criteria has both 100% sensitivity *and* specificity, some of the outcomes will be misclassified.

■ *Process by which individuals get diagnosed.* Factors including whether or not people have access to medical care, whether or not they report their symptoms to their medical provider, as well as the clinical expertise of the medical provider all can create opportunities for outcome misclassification. For example, many patients with endometriosis are often misdiagnosed as having a gastrointestinal disorder. Specialized testing and surgical procedures are needed to definitively diagnose endometriosis.[10] A patient who truly has endometriosis might not receive this diagnosis at all, or might be diagnosed with some other condition by a primary care provider who lacks the specialized knowledge and access to necessary diagnostic tests. In countries without universal healthcare insurance and access to care, there can be important associations between factors such as education, income, and race/ethnicity and whether people can access care and have their condition diagnosed.

■ *High proportion of asymptomatic cases.* Asymptomatic cases are difficult to identify without intentionally testing for their presence. A good recent example is COVID-19. Early studies during the pandemic showed that about 40% of COVID-19 cases were asymptomatic.[11] As a result, unless a highly sensitive biological test was given to everyone, individuals who were truly infected with the SARS-CoV2 virus but did not have any symptoms of infection would be misclassified as *not* having COVID-19.

■ *Patients are being effectively treated for the condition.* As discussed above, someone effectively treated for hypertension would not have high blood pressure when measured in the clinic. Or, someone effectively treated for depression would not demonstrate depressive symptoms measured by the Beck Depression Inventory. When treatment is highly effective, the symptoms of the disease are unlikely to present, and other ways of identifying the outcome are needed. For example, in addition to measuring blood pressure in the clinic, you also need to ask participants whether or not they take medications to treat hypertension. Or, in addition to administering the Beck Depression Inventory, you also need to ask participants whether or not they take medications to treat depression. And, some effectively treated diabetics will have normal glucose and HbA1c levels and consider themselves not to have diabetes, even though they are regularly taking medications to treat their diabetes.

■ *Disease is defined differently across its natural history.* Many chronic diseases are in fact a spectrum of earlier and/or less severe disease up to later stage, invasive disease that is debilitating and perhaps even causes death. The conclusions you can draw from a study depend on exactly how the outcome is defined. In other words, risk factors for *diagnosis* of a particular cancer could be different from the risk factors for *death* from that same cancer. If you define your outcome groups too narrowly, you might have fewer cases and thus lower statistical power and greater imprecision in your effect estimates. However, if you define your outcome too broadly, you could increase the potential for bias in your estimates by including

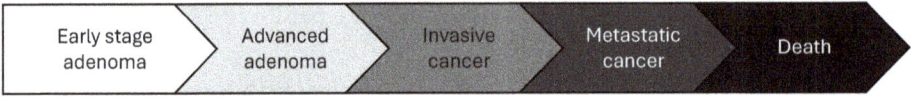

| Early stage adenoma | Advanced adenoma | Invasive cancer | Metastatic cancer | Death |

Figure 7.3 Outcome misclassification can occur due to how the outcome is defined relative to the natural history of disease, as shown in this example of the natural history of colorectal cancer.

dissimilar subgroups of the outcome. This is especially problematic if certain sub-groups of the disease are related to the exposure under study. You also should note that your scientific understanding of diseases evolves over time, which may also affect how it is classified. For example, "breast cancer" historically was considered a single outcome, but in recent decades molecular technology has evolved and led to the identification of various subtypes, which are recognized as distinct diseases with potentially different etiologies.

As an example, let's consider the natural history of colorectal cancer (Figure 7.3). Researchers have established that 10–20 years occur between the initiating events that cause early stage adenomas that, if left untreated, can progress to advanced adenoma, invasive and then metastatic cancer, and ultimately death. If you defined a study's outcome as anyone with an abnormal finding on a colonoscopy, then you would be considering early stage adenomas (as well as benign colon polyps) as essentially equivalent to invasive colorectal cancer. On the other hand, if you define your outcome as death due to colorectal cancer, you would be considering indi-viduals with adenomas or diagnosed invasive/metastatic disease as not having the outcome. And, if you define your outcome as presence of early stage adenomas, you would need to give everyone in the study a colonoscopy to avoid misclassification—because early stage adenomas are typically asymptomatic, their presence would be unknown to patients and medical providers unless they are all screened. If oppor-tunity or acceptance of screening is associated with the exposure under study, this could potentially cause differential misclassification of outcome.

When I read an article, how do I evaluate outcome misclassification?

As you read an article, you will want to pay close attention to how the outcome is measured. This should be described thoroughly in the Methods section, and many articles will create a sub-section specifically for describing the outcome assessment. Remember—there is no definitive test for outcome misclassification. However, consid-ering the following questions as you read the article can help to identify strengths and limitations of the outcome assessment and evaluate their impact on internal validity:

- *Do investigators use a standard definition for what constitutes an outcome? Is their definition strict enough to prevent misclassification?*
- *Is the outcome defined broadly or narrowly with respect to the natural history of the disease or condition under study?*
- *Has the outcome measurement been validated against a gold standard? If so, what is its sensitivity and specificity?*

- *Is the outcome measurement reliable?*
- *Were the same methods used to assess outcomes in exposed and unexposed groups?*
- *Were those making the diagnosis aware of the participant's exposure status?*
- *What is the diagnostic process for identifying the outcome? Are there reasons (e.g., access to specialized care, health insurance status, etc.) that this process would differ across groups of participants, especially those defined by exposure status?*
- *Does the process used to identify outcomes reflect an understanding of the disease/condition itself (e.g., investigators seeking to identify cases of hypertension would need to rely on more than just clinical blood pressure measurements, since people can be effectively treated for hypertension—they may no longer be symptomatic and have high blood pressure, but they would still be considered as having hypertension)?*
- *Could the exposure have affected the chances of being diagnosed?*

Additionally, similar to exposure assessment, you can review the results reported in an article to help us assess the potential for error and bias in the outcome measurement. As you read through the Results and examine the tables, considering the following questions can be helpful:

- *Do the reported associations between other factors (e.g., age, education, known risk factors) and the outcome match what you would expect based on prior studies?*
- *Does the study provide results of analyses intended to examine the impact of potential sources of bias (e.g., repeating analyses excluding self-reported outcomes that could not be verified through medical records), and, if so, are the results of these analyses similar to those of the primary analyses?*
- *Have the investigators attempted to validate their outcome ascertainment in a subset of participants? If so, did this sub-study demonstrate their outcome assessment to be valid?*
- *How do results change when different measures of the outcome are used (e.g., self-report vs medical records) or when different classifications of the outcome are used (e.g., including all cases of the outcome vs examining disease subtypes)?*

STAR in action: examining the outcome in Mirick et al.

Table 7.2 shows how we can use the STAR template to critically assess the outcome measurement approach used in a study, using the Mirick et al.[12] article as an example.

The outcome of interest is breast cancer, with cases identified through the cancer registry at the Fred Hutchinson Cancer Research Center. This is a highly valid approach for identifying cases, given that all breast cancer cases diagnosed within the hospital's catchment area would be identified and extensive diagnostic data are available on the cases. Differential misclassification of outcome is not a concern, as it is highly unlikely that case ascertainment would be at all influenced by whether or not individuals used antiperspirants/deodorants. Additionally, non-differential misclassification of outcome is of very minimal concern given that high validity of the cancer registry. There is a small chance that women identified as controls (i.e., not having breast cancer), could have undetected and undiagnosed breast cancer. However, given

Table 7.2 Completed STAR template section 4: "Outcome Assessment" for Mirick et al. (2002)[12]

Outcome assessment	
Describe (i.e., report just the facts described in the article)	Critique (i.e., think through strengths/limitations of the methods and results; address the key questions listed, and add additional comments as needed)
What was the primary outcome of interest? **Breast cancer**	Is this outcome appropriate for addressing the stated objective? **Yes, matches the stated research question.**
How was the primary outcome measured? Be specific—include details of measurement tools, assays, etc. used. **Cases were identified via cancer registry at Fred Hutchinson Cancer Research Center.** **Cases were diagnosed between November 1992 and March 1995 with International Classification of Diseases for Oncology (ICD-O) codes 174.0–174.9**	Was the measurement of outcome reliable? Was the measurement of outcome valid? What strengths and/or limitations do you note? **Yes, using a cancer registry as listed above is a reliable and valid measurement to identify cases of breast cancer; this approach is less likely to be susceptible to bias or error. Cancer registry covers geographic area from which source population is derived.** Could the study results have been affected by **differential** misclassification of outcome? Why or why not? If so, describe direction, magnitude, and likelihood. **Unlikely; differential misclassification could have occurred if those who use antiperspirant/deodorant are more likely to be screened for breast cancer and then diagnosed than those who did not report using those products. Because this scenario seems unlikely, differential misclassification of outcome would not have an important impact on study results.** Could the study results have been affected by **nondifferential** misclassification of the outcome? Why or why not? If so, describe direction, magnitude and likelihood. **Non-differential misclassification is less likely to occur in this study since they used a validated cancer registry. Although there is always a very minor chance that a participant could have been misdiagnosed or there was a systematic error with the database. It also seems very unlikely that there would have been underdiagnosed disease among controls. This again is unlikely to occur or have a notable impact on the study results.** Note any additional comments: **Overall, a very strong outcome assessment**

that mammography utilization is quite high among U.S. women, this is less likely. Non-differential misclassification of outcome is anticipated to have a minimal impact on the study's results. The highly valid approach to outcome assessment is a particular strength of the Mirick et al. study.

Activities

Find a recently published observational study or randomized controlled trial on a topic of interest to you. You might consider using the article you read for the Activities from Chapter 6.

1. Complete Section 4 of the STAR template for this article to describe how the outcome was measured and evaluate the potential for bias and error.
2. Based on your answers to the questions in the STAR template, evaluate how the outcome assessment affects the internal validity of the study.
3. Think about other approaches to outcome assessment for the outcome of interest in the article. How might these other approaches serve to either strengthen or limit internal validity? Would these approaches be more or less feasible, given the study design and study population under study in the article?

References

1. Sington JD, Cottrell BJ. Analysis of the sensitivity of death certificates in 440 hospital deaths: A comparison with necropsy findings. *J Clin Pathol.* 2002;55(7):499–502.
2. PubMed. PubMed. Accessed August 13, 2024. https://pubmed.ncbi.nlm.nih.gov
3. Home Page | United States Preventive Services Taskforce. Accessed August 13, 2024. https://www.uspreventiveservicestaskforce.org/uspstf/
4. Cochrane. Accessed August 13, 2024. https://www.cochrane.org/evidence
5. UpToDate: Trusted, Evidence-Based Solutions for Modern Healthcare. Accessed August 13, 2024. https://www.wolterskluwer.com/en/solutions/uptodate
6. Hart V, Sturgeon SR, Reich N, et al. Menopausal vasomotor symptoms and incident breast cancer risk in the study of women's health across the nation. *Cancer Causes Control.* 2016;27(11):1333–1340. doi:10.1007/s10552-016-0811-9
7. National Lung Screening Trial Research Team, Church TR, Black WC, et al. Results of initial low-dose computed tomographic screening for lung cancer. *N Engl J Med.* 2013;368(21):1980–1991. doi:10.1056/NEJMoa1209120
8. Lash TL, VanderWeele TJ, Haneuse S, Rothman KJ, eds. *Modern Epidemiology.* 4th edition. Wolters Kluwer; 2021.
9. Celentano D, Szklo M, Farag Y. Gordis Epidemiology. 7th edition. Elsevier; 2024.
10. Greene R, Stratton P, Cleary SD, Ballweg ML, Sinaii N. Diagnostic experience among 4,334 women reporting surgically diagnosed endometriosis. *Fertil Steril.* 2009;91(1):32–39. doi:10.1016/j.fertnstert.2007.11.020
11. Oran DP, Topol EJ. Prevalence of asymptomatic SARS-CoV-2 infection : A narrative review. *Ann Intern Med.* 2020;173(5):362–367. doi:10.7326/M20–3012
12. Mirick DK, Davis S, Thomas DB. Antiperspirant use and the risk of breast cancer. *J Natl Cancer Inst.* 2002;94(20):1578–1580. doi:10.1093/jnci/94.20.1578

CHAPTER 8

How were the data analyzed?

If you are like most students, you are starting this chapter with more than a little anxiety about statistics. Rest assured, this chapter will not delve into theoretical details and derivations of formulae. There are plenty of excellent biostatistics textbooks that present that type of information. It is important for anyone reading epidemiologic articles to have a solid understanding of introductory (and perhaps even intermediate) biostatistics. As epidemiologists and health professionals, however, you also need to know the limits of your knowledge and when to call in an expert.

When I teach applied data analysis to epidemiology graduate students, I use this story as an analogy. I am a licensed driver, and I know a lot about how to operate my car. I know how to drive it on windy country roads, through congested city blocks, and on busy highways. I know how to fill it with gas and check the oil. But, I am not a mechanic. When the "check engine" light goes on or the brakes start squeaking, I know that I need to bring it to the service station where someone with expertise in auto mechanics can diagnose and solve the problems. And, I know just enough of the basic terminology and about how a car works that I can have a conversation with the mechanics and understand what they plan to do to fix my car. I consider myself a "knowledgeable driver."

As epidemiologists and health professionals, you need to be knowledgeable drivers of the statistical analysis—you need to understand enough to handle the basics, recognize when more expertise is needed, and be conversant enough in the details to understand what those experts are saying. Biostatisticians are the mechanics—they have both a broader and a more in-depth knowledge of statistical analyses, and you should be consulting them for their expertise as needed. As knowledgeable drivers, you need to understand what types of analyses are appropriate in various situations, but you don't necessarily need to memorize all the equations or be able to run the more sophisticated analyses yourselves.

In this chapter, we will focus on how to evaluate whether the data were analyzed appropriately and whether appropriate conclusions were drawn from the results.

DOI: 10.4324/9781003637899-9

We will discuss what statistical approaches are used in various situations, explore confounding and effect modification, and consider important questions related to whether appropriate analyses were conducted.

How do I determine when to use different statistical tests and methods?

First, you need to identify the scale of the exposure and outcome variables. Variable scale is critical for determining what statistical approach to use. In general, variables can be classified as either continuous or categorical. A **continuous variable** is one that can take on a (seemingly) infinite range of values (e.g., participant's age can be reported in years to many decimal places). **Categorical variables**, on the other hand, have a limited set of values. Often the number of a categorical variable gives information (e.g., providing pain symptoms on a scale of 0–10). In some cases, though, these values aren't numeric but rather classify participants into groups based on a characteristic that has no inherent ordering (e.g., race, ethnicity, gender, geographic location). Any time you are using data to put participants into groups, you are using a categorical variable.

Table 8.1 shows the most common statistical approaches used for different combinations of variable scales for the exposure and outcome. Of these two key variables, the outcome variable's scale is typically more important in determining the statistical analysis approach that needs to be used.

Imagine that you want to explore an association between age (our exposure) and body mass index (BMI, your outcome). If you measure both your exposure (e.g., age, measured in years) and your outcome (e.g., BMI, measured in kg/m^2) as continuous variables, you could test for an association between them by calculating a correlation coefficient. However, if you decided to categorize BMI into two groups (e.g., below the median or

Table 8.1 The choice of statistical approach is determined by the scale of the exposure and outcome variables. The table lists the most common statistical approaches used in epidemiologic studies by scale of the exposure (independent) and outcome (dependent) variables

		Outcome (dependent variable)	
		Continuous	*Categorical*
Exposure (independent variable)	**Continuous**	■ Correlation coefficient ■ Linear regression	■ t-test (for 2 groups) ■ Analysis of variance (ANOVA) (for 2+ groups) ■ Logistic regression (for binary outcome) ■ Cox proportional hazards regression (for binary outcome with time-to-event data)
	Categorical	■ t-test (for 2 groups) ■ ANOVA (for 2+ groups) ■ Linear regression	■ Chi-square test ■ Logistic regression (for binary outcome) ■ Cox proportional hazards regression (for binary outcome with time-to-event data)

at/above the median), you would instead test whether mean age is different between the two BMI groups using a two-sample t-test. Or, if you decided to categorize BMI using the World Health Organization's cutpoints (underweight/normal [<25 kg/m^2], overweight [25–<30 kg/m^2]), and obese [≥30 kg/m^2]), you would need to use analysis of variance (ANOVA) to test to differences in mean age across the three BMI categories (since ANOVA is used to assess differences in means across two or more groups). In each case, the exposure variable (age) is the same, but how the outcome variable is represented (BMI) changes, and thus the statistical test to be used changes as well.

What are the most common regression approaches used in epidemiologic studies?

Regression approaches have the advantage of facilitating estimation of measures of association that are adjusted by one or more other variables. For this reason, they are used extensively in epidemiologic studies. With regression approaches, you would use linear regression when the outcome variable is continuous (e.g., continuous BMI) or you would use logistic regression when the outcome variable is binary (e.g., underweight/normal vs overweight/obese) and Cox proportional hazards regression when the outcome variable is binary and also includes time-to-event data. All three regression approaches can incorporate continuous and categorical independent variables.

Linear regression

Linear regression is similar to the equation for a straight line we all learned about in middle school: $y = mx + b$. Now that we are older and presumably smarter, we represent this same equation using Greek letters: $y = \beta_0 + \beta_1 x$. The association between exposure (x) and outcome (y) is estimated through the β coefficient for the exposure (β_1), which estimates the change in outcome (y) per every one unit change in exposure (x) (i.e., β_1 is the slope of the line—what our teenage selves would have denoted as m). As additional variables are added to the linear regression model, each β coefficient is adjusted for the other variables in the model. For example, a multivariable linear regression model was fit to estimate longitudinal associations between BMI and mammographic density, showing that for each 1-unit increase in BMI, mammographic density decreased by 1.17% (95% CI –1.31 to –1.04).[1]

Logistic regression

Logistic regression requires a binary outcome variable and facilitates the estimation of the odds ratio (OR). Case-control studies quite naturally use logistic regression for analyzing their data, since the outcome can have only one of two values (i.e., case or control). As variables are added (e.g., confounders) to the logistic regression model, the resulting OR estimate for the exposure of interest is adjusted for the other variables in the model. I will spare you the theoretical details here, but you should know the β coefficient for an independent variable in a logistic regression model is interpretable as the ln(OR) for a one-unit change in that variable. You can calculate the OR for that variable as OR = e^β. Happily, most statistical analysis programs will calculate this for you, and most epidemiologic articles will report the ORs (not the coefficients). For example, a recent study performed a logistic regression analysis to show that pregnant females who had at least two virtual appointments with a doula during their pregnancy had a 20% reduction in odds of cesarean section births (OR 0.80, 95% CI 0.65–0.99).[2]

Cox proportional hazards regression

A third regression approach that is commonly used in epidemiologic studies is **Cox proportional hazards regression**. Follow-up studies (i.e., prospective cohort studies and randomized controlled trials) have information on both the outcome (i.e., whether or not outcome occurred during follow-up) and the length of time participants were followed. In other words, the outcome is more than just a binary variable and requires an approach that can account for the person-time each participant contributes to the study. Cox proportional hazards regression is also referred to as "survival analysis." Cox models can be used to estimate the hazard ratio (HR, a.k.a. the relative risk or risk ratio) as a measure of the association between exposure and outcome, taking into account varying amounts of follow-up time for the study participants. As in linear and logistic regression models, additional variables can be added to the Cox proportional hazards regression model such that the HRs estimated are adjusted for potential confounding from the other variables included in the model. For example, a recent prospective cohort study in Denmark reported a substantially increased risk of endometrial cancer among women with polycystic ovary syndrome (HR 3.02, 95% CI 2.03–4.49).[3]

How should I think about statistical power?

Recall that statistical power refers to the ability to detect that an association exists (i.e., to reject the null hypothesis), given that there is truly an association between the variables under study (i.e., given that the null hypothesis is false). When reading an epidemiologic article, it is important to consider whether the sample size provided sufficient statistical power for testing the stated hypotheses.

It is especially important to consider whether statistical power was sufficient when the study reports a "null" result. Imagine a case-control study of 75 cases and 75 matched controls that reports an OR = 1.6 (95% CI 0.8–2.5) as their primary result. Given the small sample size and the CI that is suggesting a trend toward a positive association, we should rightly question whether the study had sufficient statistical power for testing their null hypothesis. It is certainly possible that a much larger study might have had sufficient statistical power to reject the null hypothesis given the same OR estimate of 1.6.

You might note that epidemiologic articles often don't report their level of statistical power in their published manuscripts. Even if the statistical power isn't stated, you could calculate it yourself by inputting their results into one of the many handy online power calculators (just search "statistical power calculator" using your favorite search tool and pick one hosted by a reputable university). You also should develop a sense for when power might be insufficient based on sample size (e.g., case-control studies with <100 cases, prospective cohort studies with <100 outcomes) or the association to be detected (e.g., small associations such as OR = 1.1 or a difference in means of 0.1).

What is the problem with multiple comparisons?

If you perform a statistical test at $\alpha = 0.05$, there is a 5% chance that you will incorrectly reject the null hypothesis. In other words, out of every twenty statistical tests, on average one will be statistically significant by chance alone. It is logical, then, to recognize that the more statistical tests are performed, the greater chance there is that one of them is a Type I error; this phenomenon is often referred to as an issue of **multiple comparisons**. In fact, the Type I error rate actually increases more than you might have guessed. For n statistical tests performed at a given α, the effective Type I error rate, which you'll denote as α^*, is actually: $\alpha^* = 1-(1-\alpha)^n$. So, if you perform a series of six pairwise comparisons at $\alpha = 0.05$, your effective Type I error rate is $\alpha^* = 1-(1-0.05)^6 = 0.265$. It's ok if you don't remember the math here, as long as you remember this: the more statistical tests have been performed, the greater the chance that at least one represents a Type I error.

Often, studies will employ statistical approaches (e.g., Bonferroni correction) that address the multiple comparisons issue and preserve the overall Type I error rate at the desired level. If such methods are not described in their statistical analysis methods description, then you should consider the potential impact of Type I error on the reported results. When you read an epidemiologic article, if the study has performed, for example, thirty different statistical tests and only one shows up as significant, you should question if that is perhaps reflecting a Type I error as opposed to a true association. This is especially true if that single statistically significant result seems inconsistent with other results reported in the paper. For example, an analysis to evaluate whether consumption of coffee and tea was associated with risk of melanoma[4] observed overwhelmingly null results, indicating no association between coffee/tea and melanoma risk. However, a single, statistically significant positive association was observed between drinking two or more cups of tea each day and melanoma (HR 1.36, 95% CI 1.00–1.84). Because this was the only statistically significant result among the many analyses, and because none of the other results indicated any meaningful association between coffee or tea consumption and melanoma risk, the authors concluded that this statistically significant association was likely to be a Type I error, rather than reflecting a true, causal association.

What is the problem with missing data?

First, let's talk about what missing data is and why it matters. Simply put, **missing data** refers to when a participant lacks data on one of the variables included in the analysis. The variable could be the exposure, the outcome, or some other variable such as a covariate. Missing data can be missing for any number of reasons: the participant wasn't asked the question, the participant didn't want to answer the question, the question didn't apply to the participant, etc.

Most of the time epidemiologists assume that the missing data are **missing completely at random**. In other words, we assume that there is no relationship between the participant's *actual* value for the missing data (if we could know it) and the fact that they are missing data for that variable; we also assume there is no relationship between missingness in the variable and the values of other variables, including those of the exposure, outcome, or other covariates. For example, if missing data in a study occur because a page was missing from the questionnaire for some participants, and the incomplete questionnaires were randomly distributed among the participants, then we could safely say that the data are missing completely at random. In reality, this is a very strong assumption.

Much of the time, however, missing data are *not* missing completely at random. There are often known or unknown reasons why participants would have missing data. Imagine that you ask a group of participants to report their annual family income. Many participants will not want to report how much they earn, and there will be a lot of missing data for this variable as a result. It is very likely that those participants who don't provide an answer to a question about their income differ in important ways from those who do respond. For example, one study found that those missing income data on a survey had sociodemographic characteristics that were more similar to those known to have lower incomes as opposed to those known to have higher incomes.[5]

An important problem with missing data arises when it causes participants to be excluded from the analysis. If a participant is missing data for a variable that is included in the statistical analysis (e.g., missing data on income in a linear regression that includes income as a confounder), then that participant is not included in the analytic sample. Statistical analysis programs automatically drop any observations with missing values for the variables specified in the statistical test; this is often referred to as **complete case analysis**. At a minimum, dropping these participants from the statistical analysis will decrease the sample size and thus decrease the statistical power. But if missingness is not completely at random (which, in reality, it generally isn't), then bias can result. This is a sneaky way for selection bias to occur. Based on the recruitment procedures described, you might have decided that there was no evidence of selection bias in the study. But, if there are a lot of missing data that cause some participants to be dropped from the analysis, and if the missingness is somehow related to exposure and outcome status, you now have selection bias.

Imagine a hypothetical study of an association between annual family income and risk of Parkinson's disease using data from a prospective cohort (Figure 8.1). If you had complete data on all participants, you would see that there is truly no association between income level and risk of Parkinson's disease (RR = 1.0; Figure 8.1A). However, some participants are missing data on their annual family income and are not included in the analysis. In this extreme example, the participants missing income data are low income and diagnosed with Parkinson's disease during follow-up (Figure 8.1B). Based on the non-missing participants, you would incorrectly conclude that high-income individuals are nearly twice as likely as low-income individuals to be diagnosed with Parkinson's disease (RR = 1.9).

Fortunately, there are ways to address missing data in statistical analyses. Multiple imputation is a statistical approach that is commonly used to "fill in" the missing data by using a statistical model to essentially make an educated guess about what the participant's value for the missing data would be if that had reported it. I will spare you a lengthy discussion of the math behind multiple imputation and other approaches to analytically addressing missing data issues. Those who are interested in digging deeper into this topic can find many great references (e.g., *Statistical Analysis with Missing Data* by Little and Rubin[6]).

Suffice it to say that you should pay attention to how missing data are addressed when you read journal articles. Often, researchers will note where missing data occur and describe how they handled it analytically. But sometimes they are far less transparent.

A. Study Population

	Parkinson's Disease	No Parkinson's Disease	
High Income	100	900	1000
Low Income	100	900	1000

RR= (100/1000) / (100/1000) = 1.0

B. Analytic Population

	Parkinson's Disease	No Parkinson's Disease	
High Income	100	900	1000
Low Income	50	900	950

RR= (100/1000) / (50/950) = 1.9

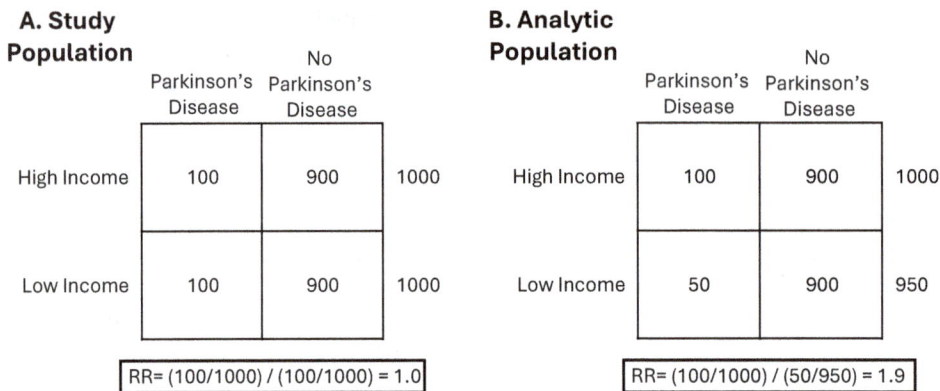

Figure 8.1 Selection bias can arise when missing data are related to exposure and outcome and participants with missing data are excluded from analyses. In this hypothetical extreme example, investigators examine an association between income and Parkinson's disease among 2,000 participants in a prospective cohort study. If all participants in the study population could be included in the analysis, (A. Study Population), no association between income and Parkinson's disease would be observed. However, 50 participants are missing data on income, and (in reality) they are low income and diagnosed with Parkinson's disease (B. Analytic Population). A selection bias occurs, and the estimated relative risk indicates a positive association between income and Parkinson's disease.

You should pay particular attention to how the analytic sample changes as a result of missing data. Often, you can detect these changes by paying careful attention to the sample size (often represented as **N**) that contributes to the analysis, which is often provided in the tables. If you notice that the N changes for the actual analysis, you should question why. You also should consider whether the missing data might have resulted in a selection bias that would affect the internal validity of the study's results.

What is confounding?

You probably remember from your introductory epidemiology course that a **confounder** is a third factor that affects the apparent association between the exposure and outcome being studied. Hopefully, you also remember that the confounding factor is one that is: (1) non-causally associated with the exposure, (2) causally associated with the outcome, and (3) not on the causal pathway linking the exposure to the outcome.

A good example of confounding is to consider the crude overall mortality rate in the U.S. states of Utah (647.4 deaths per 100,000 per year) and Florida (1,074.9 deaths per 100,000 per year). At first glance, you might wonder what is going on in Florida that its mortality rate is so much higher than Utah's. But, Florida residents tend to be older than Utah residents, and older people are more likely to die. Given these two facts, you can recognize that age is acting as a confounder of the association between state of residence and all-cause mortality. In fact, when the mortality rates are adjusted for age, you see that the age-adjusted all-cause mortality rates are actually quite similar for the two states (755.0 vs 714.0 deaths per 100,000 per year for Utah and Florida, respectively).[7]

Let's take our discussion of confounding a step further and think about counterfactuals to help us understand how confounding arises. This is a big word that might feel intimidating. But, my guess is that you already have an inherent sense of what a counterfactual scenario is and how it relates to confounding. Put simply, a **counterfactual** is a condition that is impossible to directly observe. If you really wanted to know whether an exposure is related to an outcome, you would ideally compare what happens to the *same* person when they are exposed versus when they are unexposed. This is just not possible when studying humans, though. If you are studying animals, you could design an experiment with genetically similar animals that are kept in similar living conditions (e.g., housing, food, socialization) and then expose one group but not the other. However, you cannot do this with your human participants. When you study humans, you can observe what happens following the exposure (or lack of exposure), but you cannot directly observe the counterfactual scenario. In other words, you cannot see what happens to the same exact person under the opposite exposure status.

Epidemiologic studies are built around the idea of having comparison groups that can represent the counterfactual scenario as closely as possible. But this can never be done perfectly, because patterns of exposure are not randomly distributed throughout the population. Other characteristics including age, race/ethnicity, geographic location, and many behavioral choices can impact exposure status. When those characteristics are non-causally associated with exposure and causally associated with outcome, you have confounding.

The effects of a confounder on the observed association between exposure and outcome can be to bias the estimate either away from or toward the null. To figure out in which direction the bias is going, you need to consider each scenario individually. The direction of the confounding effect will depend on the direction of the confounder's association with exposure and outcome. An in-depth discussion of how confounding alters the effect estimate is beyond the scope of this text, but I can refer you to some great resources on this topic.[8,9]

Also, results may still be affected by confounding, even when appropriate methods have been used to attempt to control confounders. This idea is often referred to as **residual confounding**, and it exists because we cannot ever observe the counterfactual scenario. Even if studies address confounding in their design and/or analysis, residual confounding can still be present as a result of: (1) unknown confounders, (2) unmeasured confounders, or (3) confounders that have imprecision and/or misclassification in their measurements. For example, a study that adjusts for age by grouping people into 10-year age intervals can still have residual confounding by age. There is quite a biologic difference between, say, a 41-year-old and a 49-year-old, even though they would both be included in a 40–49-year-old age group. Adjusting for age by smaller age intervals would provide more complete adjustment for confounding by age and minimize the potential for residual confounding.

How do investigators control for confounding when designing and analyzing the study?

Researchers can address confounding when they are designing the study and when they are analyzing the data. Many studies will use a combination of these approaches. While various methods to control for confounders exist, you probably expect by now that each method comes with its own set of strengths and limitations (like pretty much everything else in epidemiology). And you'd be right! Let's take a closer look at five general approaches to addressing confounding: matching, restriction, randomization, stratification, and multivariable regression.

Matching

Individual matching is a common form of controlling for confounding in case-control studies. In these contexts, matching means that for each case enrolled, one (or more than one) control is enrolled that matches the case on a pre-determined set of characteristics. Common matching factors include age, race/ethnicity, and sex assigned at birth. For example, investigators conducted a matched case-control study to evaluate associations between mobile phone use and brain tumors in children and adolescents, where controls were individually matched to cases on age, geographic location, and date of diagnosis.[10]

An important strength of matching is that it can provide excellent control for confounding. The reason why is fairly obvious: we have ensured that cases and their matched control(s) have the same values for the confounders that were used as matching factors (e.g., a male case is matched with a male control, so there is no variability between cases and controls with respect to sex).

There are some limitations associated with individual matching, however. First, residual confounding can still occur if the matching is imperfect or if the range for an allowable match is too wide (e.g., if matching on age is done ±5 years, then there could be residual confounding by age). Second, matching on specific criteria at the design phase precludes an ability to investigate these factors during analysis. For example, a case-control study with matching done on race/ethnicity would be unable to evaluate whether race/ethnicity is associated with the outcome. Third, it can be challenging to find controls that are exact matches for the cases, and you would need to collect information on the matching factors before enrolling the controls into the study. All this leads to logistical and timing issues that ultimately make recruitment take longer and cost more.

Here, we need to distinguish between individual matching (what I've just described) and **frequency matching.** In frequency matched studies, investigators aim to enroll a control group that has similar overall prevalence of certain characteristics as the case group. Frequency matching does not control for confounding but rather is done to enhance comparability and efficiency of the study population. For example, the Long Island Breast Cancer Study Project frequency matched breast cancer cases and controls by 5-year age group.[11]

Restriction

Another approach to controlling for confounding in the design of the study is to **restrict** the study population to those with (or without) presence of the confounder. Oftentimes this is done because the association between the confounder and outcome is so strong that it could mask smaller associations with the exposure of interest (e.g., restricting to non-smokers in a study of radon exposure and lung cancer). For example, a study evaluating associations between circulating hormone levels and breast cancer restricted analysis to include only those participants not currently using postmenopausal hormone therapy, given its strong potential for confounding.[12]

A clear strength of this approach is that it eliminates any potential confounding effects by the restriction factor, assuming the restriction is done appropriately. However, a limitation is that the restriction factor cannot be evaluated for potential effect modification since there is no variability in the restriction factor (e.g., you couldn't evaluate if smoking status modifies an association if you are only studying non-smokers). Additionally, restricting the study population in the design phase based on presence or absence of a given factor means that future studies within the same study population cannot consider that factor in their analysis either. Also, such restrictions may decrease the external validity of the study.

Randomization

Perhaps the most effective approach to adjust for confounding is **randomization**. Randomization means that participants don't select their own exposure groups, but rather are assigned through a random process (e.g., a flip of a coin). Assuming sufficient numbers of participants, randomization to exposed and unexposed groups will create balance on confounders, both known and unknown, between the groups. For example, a randomized controlled trial assigned participants to follow either their regular diet or the Dietary Approaches to Stop Hypertension (DASH) diet.[13] The randomization resulted in groups that had similar distributions of potential confounding factors, including age (49 yrs vs 47 yrs, respectively) and race (56% vs 57% Black).

While this approach offers important strengths, its limitations should be obvious as well. Randomization is not a possibility for observational studies. And, as was discussed in Chapter 4, experimental designs are frequently impractical, unethical, or otherwise infeasible for epidemiologic studies.

Stratification

Stratification is an approach that can be implemented in the analysis phase by repeating analyses within subgroups defined by the confounder. This is somewhat similar to restriction, except that no one is permanently excluded from the study. Instead, separate estimates of effect are calculated within each stratum (e.g., estimating the effect of radon on lung cancer risk among non-smokers and separately among smokers). Because everyone in the stratum has the same value for the confounder, the estimated associations within each stratum are unaffected by confounding from that particular factor. For example, a study of genital powder use and endometrial cancer risk stratified by BMI, given strong potential for confounding by BMI.[14]

Strengths of this approach are very similar to those of restriction. The confounding bias from a particular factor is removed within the strata, provided that the strata are appropriately defined and have minimal misclassification. Continuing the example of radon and lung cancer, confounding by smoking is eliminated within the two strata (i.e., non-smokers and smokers), provided that there is no misclassification in measuring smoking status. An advantage of stratification compared to restriction, though, is that the participants all remain in the study population and in the analytic population.

Additionally, the confounding factor still can be examined for effect modification, or as the exposure of interest in future studies.

An important limitation is that, depending on the distribution of the confounder in the study population, some strata may have small sample sizes, leading to imprecision in effect estimates. For example, if your study population included only five lung cancer cases among non-smokers, you would not be able to calculate a precise estimate of the association between radon and lung cancer among non-smokers.

Multivariable regression

Perhaps the most common approach to adjusting for confounding is to include the confounder as a variable in the regression model that is fit to estimate the association between exposure and outcome. While the other approaches to addressing confounding typically can adjust for only one or two confounders simultaneously, **multivariable regression** models can provide statistical adjustment for confounding for multiple variables all at one time. For example, an analysis of depression and breast cancer risk used multivariable regression to simultaneously adjust for many confounders, including age, BMI, and physical activity.[15] The ability to control for multiple confounders at once is a key strength of multivariable regression models. A limitation, however, is that smaller studies may have insufficient numbers to allow for more than a few confounders to be included in the regression model while still maintaining good precision of the estimated associations.

When I read an article, how do I assess confounding?

Even if you fully understand confounding and can identify ways to address it when designing and analyzing your own studies, it can be challenging to think through the presence and implications of confounding when you read epidemiologic articles. Recognizing whether confounders were identified and appropriately controlled for is an important component of your critical analysis. As you read the methods and the results of these studies, asking yourself some pointed questions can be helpful:

■ *Are well-established confounders considered and addressed?* These could be identified based on prior studies evaluating associations between the exposure and outcome under study. For example, smoking has been consistently identified as a confounder of the association between alcohol and heart disease; if a study of this association does not address potential confounding by smoking, you'd (rightly) be concerned about the validity of the study's result.

■ *What other factors are considered as possible confounders?* Importantly, are there factors that could be confounders in the study population, but that have not been identified as confounders in other populations? For example, in U.S. populations, health insurance status (as a proxy for access to healthcare) is a confounder of many exposure-outcome associations. However, in countries with universal healthcare access, health insurance status would not be a confounder.

■ *How valid and precise are the measurements of the confounders?* As described above, misclassification or imprecision in the measurements can result in residual confounding. For example, adjusting for age grouped in 10-year intervals will likely have residual confounding by age.

■ *Could the study have over-adjusted by controlling for factors that are not truly confounders?* Think through the causal pathway—has the study adjusted for factors that are either on the causal pathway or that are influenced by both exposure and outcome? Doing so also will lead to invalid study results. For example, you would not want to adjust for hypertension in a study exploring associations between dietary sodium intake and heart disease, because dietary sodium intake leads to hypertension which then leads to heart disease.

You might be wondering how you can possibly answer the above questions. I'll admit that it isn't always (or ever?) easy. But, you can start with a careful reading of the Methods section, especially the statistical analysis sub-section, as well as carefully reading any footnotes included in the results tables. Look for any eligibility criteria that might be seeking to control confounding through restriction (e.g., excluding current smokers). Determine whether matching was used and, if so, on what variables. See what variables the researchers consider as they build a multi-variable model—are they missing some factors that you think should have been included? Are they including some factors that you know to be an intermediate step in their hypothesized causal pathway? How have they measured, defined, and categorized these factors? Is there any misclassification in the measurement of these factors? After you carefully read through a few statistical analysis sub-sections, it will become easier to identify how confounding was addressed and if those approaches were sufficient (trust me).

What is effect modification?

In all my years of teaching epidemiology, effect modification is easily the concept that confuses students the most (with selection bias coming in as a close second). It's a challenging concept, but I've found that the most effective way to help students understand it is with two simple words: "it depends."

To provide a formal definition, **effect modification** is when the association between exposure and outcome is different across levels of a third factor. In other words, the causal association between exposure and outcome *depends* on the level of this third factor. When effect modification is present, if you want to describe the association between exposure and outcome, you will have to say "it depends" on the value of this third factor.

Here's a real-life example, based on dozens of epidemiologic research studies. Obesity (the exposure) has a different association with breast cancer (the outcome) depending on the woman's menopausal status (the third factor) (Figure 8.2). Specifically, among postmenopausal women, obesity (defined as BMI ≥30 kg/m^2) increases breast cancer risk by about 30% compared to normal-weight women.[16] However, among premenopausal women, obesity is associated with about 30% lower breast cancer risk compared to normal-weight women.[17] So if anyone asks you what the association between obesity and breast cancer is, you would have to answer that "it depends" on menopausal status.

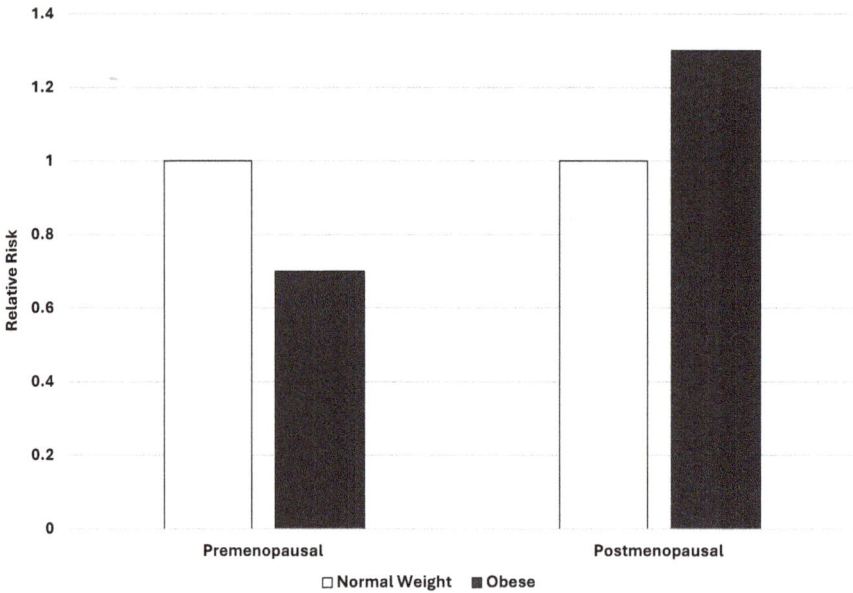

Figure 8.2 Effect modification occurs when the association between an exposure and outcome differs across levels of a third variable. A well-established example of effect modification is that the association between obesity and breast cancer risk is modified by menopausal status.

It is important to note that just because a third factor is acting as an effect modifier doesn't mean that it cannot also be acting as a confounder. In fact, when evaluating causal relationships between exposure and outcome, a third factor can be a confounder, an effect modifier, neither or both. I'll refer you to other texts for in-depth discussions of causal diagrams, but suffice it to say here that if you identify a factor as an effect modifier, you still can (and should in many cases) evaluate it for potential confounding effects as well, and vice versa.

Finally, I want to underscore that when you find evidence of effect modification, your goal is not to adjust it away. Instead, effect modification is an important part of the causal mechanism and can help you understand the full nature of the relationship between exposure and outcome.

When I read an article, how do I assess effect modification?

With effect modification, you are looking to see if the association between exposure and outcome differs across strata of the effect modifier. When reading journal articles, you can scan results tables to see if the effect estimates (e.g., OR, RR) are presented by stratum of a third variable. For example, a study population including both males and females may assess associations between the exposure and outcome separately in each category of biological sex. Or, a study of breast cancer might stratify on menopausal status, as this has been shown to modify associations between many exposures and breast cancer risk (e.g., obesity).

When results are presented in this way, though, how do you know if effect modification is present? An initial approach is what I call an "eyeball test," where you simply look at the numbers and decide if they seem different or not. For example, ORs of 1.5 and 3.5 seem quite different, while ORs of 1.5 and 1.7 do not. An eyeball test can be helpful initially to give you a sense of whether or not effect modification is present, but you should not base your conclusions on it. Instead, you need to utilize a statistical test, most often a **test of homogeneity**. This statistical test essentially asks the question "are the ORs (or other measures of association) within each stratum equal to one another?" If you fail to reject the null hypothesis ($p > 0.05$), you conclude that there is no evidence that the ORs are different across strata, and you can state that there is no evidence of effect modification. However, if you reject the null hypothesis ($p \leq 0.05$), you conclude that there is evidence that the ORs are different across the strata and that effect modification is present. P values from tests of homogeneity are typically labeled as $P_{interaction}$ in results tables. The exact details regarding how to fit these types of statistical models and perform tests of homogeneity are beyond the scope of this book, but you could refer to an introductory biostatistics textbook if you want a deeper explanation.

A final important point to make regarding effect modification: when there is statistical evidence for effect modification, you should always consider whether this reflects true causal pathways or if it is an artifact of the statistical model that was fit. This is where your background knowledge is important. You should carefully think through whether the proposed causal pathway reflects biological and/or social reality, or if the effect modification observed is due to the particular statistical model fit to the data. For example, there is evidence in support of a biological mechanism that explains the effect modification by menopausal status on the association between obesity and breast cancer risk (I won't bore you with the details here, but it is thought to be related to the different hormonal environments in pre- and postmenopausal women). If, for the sake of argument, you observed statistically significant effect modification by eye color on the association between obesity and breast cancer risk, you should be suspicious that this is statistical artifact. There likely is not a plausible biological (or social) explanation for why eye color would modify the effect of obesity on breast cancer risk.

What questions should I ask about the statistical analysis as I read an epidemiologic article?

As you read epidemiologic articles, pay careful attention to the statistical analysis sub-section of the Methods section. While I know it is tempting to just skim it and move on, avoid that temptation! You need to have a good understanding of what statistical analyses were performed and any decisions or assumptions that were made along the way—these can all have significant impacts on the results that were obtained. And, it is important to closely examine all tables and figures showing results along with the accompanying text. Sometimes articles will include additional results tables and figures as supplemental material available online, and you also may need to explore those as well. In general, my message to you is to take the time to carefully examine everything for yourself, don't just assume the authors have done everything correctly. Hopefully, they did, but double-checking and making your own determination is advisable nonetheless.

As you consider the statistical analysis and results sections, the STAR template will help you to focus on the overall approach used in the statistical analysis as well as whether confounding and effect modification were considered and evaluated. An in-depth examination of the statistical analysis also should consider the following questions:

- *Was there a pre-determined statistical approach, or was it a "fishing expedition"?* Ideally, the analysis approach should be driven by the research question and out-lined prior to the analysis beginning. A "fishing expedition," however, is when analyses have the appearance of having been done until a particular, statistically significant was found.

- *Does the statistical analysis match the research question and study design?* For example, is a case-control study analyzed using logistic regression, or a prospective cohort study analyzed using Cox proportional hazards regression? If an individually matched study was conducted, are appropriate statistical approaches used for these matched data (e.g., paired t-tests, conditional logistic regression)?

- *Is there sufficient statistical power?* This is especially important to consider when the results are *not* statistically significant. Could the null findings reflect a lack of power rather a true lack of association?

- *Is the impact of multiple comparisons taken into consideration?* This is especially important to consider when there appear to be many, many statistical tests per-formed. Consider whether the results could be due to a Type I error, rather than a true association.

- *Is the impact of missing data taken into consideration?* Pay close attention to how the sample size changes from the enrolled study population to the analytic study population, looking for any potential effects on statistical power or selection bias.

- *Are results accurately presented in tables and/or figures?* It is important to verify that the results presented in the tables and figures match the analyses that were described in the Methods section as well as the information provided in the text of the Results section.

- *Are the statistical tests that are performed interpreted correctly?* Each statistical test has an appropriate interpretation. For example, a t-test compares means of two groups; it would be incorrect to state that the results of a t-test led to the conclusion that the exposure increased risk of the outcome.

- *Do the authors over-emphasize P values, especially in analyses where statistical power appears to be limited?* For example, a P value of 0.06 would suggest that there is no association, but if the study had <80% power to detect the association, this conclusion might be a Type II error.

Don't forget about systematic error (i.e., bias)! In epidemiologic studies of adequate sample size, systematic error, confounding, and misclassification (all the concepts we've been discussing before this chapter) may be even more important than random error in terms of their impact on study validity. After all, if you have determined that there are major limitations with the study population, exposure assessment, and/or outcome assessment that have a strong possibility of biased results (and, therefore, poor internal validity), the results of statistical testing don't really matter—you've already decided that the study lacks internal validity.

STAR in action: examining the statistical analysis in Mirick et al.

The primary analysis of the Mirick et al.[18] article utilized multivariable conditional logistic regression to calculate adjusted ORs. This is an appropriate statistical approach for calculating multivariable-adjusted ORs from a matched case-control study. The regression model incorporated the matching variables through the conditional logistic regression. Additional confounding variables were adjusted for in the multivariable model including important potential confounders such as parity, oral contraceptive use, family history of breast cancer, BMI, and physical activity. While no effect modifiers were evaluated in the research article, it would have been appropriate to have explored potential effect modification by menopausal status, given the known differences in pre- and postmenopausal breast cancer.

The study included a large sample size (for a case-control study), with 813 cases and 793 controls enrolled. While the article did not report its statistical power, we can use their reported findings and our favorite statistical software to calculate that this sample size afforded them 80% power to detect an OR = 1.24 as statistically significant with two-sided α = 0.05 (Table 8.2).

Table 8.2 Completed STAR template section 5: "Statistical Analysis" for Mirick et al. (2002)[18]

5. Statistical analysis	
Describe (i.e., report just the facts described in the article)	Critique (i.e., think through strengths/limitations of the methods and results; address the key questions listed, and add additional comments as needed)
What statistical analyses were performed? **Calculated adjusted odds ratios and 95% confidence intervals using multivariable logistic regression models**	Is the analytic approach appropriate for testing the specified hypotheses? Why or why not? **Yes, since this is a case-control study it is appropriate to use an odds ratio to estimate the relative risk. Also, conditional logistic regression is an appropriate statistical approach for calculating multivariable-adjusted odds ratios in a matched case-control study**
How was confounding addressed and controlled? (include both approaches in how the study was designed and how data were analyzed) Describe the important confounders that were considered. **Fit conditional multivariable logistic regression models to adjust for age through matched design and other potential confounders; identified confounders based on prior research including parity, age at first birth,**	Were these approaches sufficient to control for confounding? What is the likelihood of residual confounding? Should the authors have considered the effect of other variables not included in the study? **Yes, these approaches were appropriate for controlling for confounding. Some confounders not considered/adjusted for include body mass index and physical activity; small potential for residual confounding.**

(Continued)

Table 8.2 (*Continued*)

5. *Statistical analysis*	
first-degree family history of breast cancer, oophorectomy status, use of oral contraceptives, use of hormone therapy, use of alcohol, smoking history	
What, if any, effect modification was evaluated? None	Were the methods to evaluate effect modification sufficient? Why or why not? **Given known differences in pre- and postmenopausal breast cancer, consideration of menopausal status as an effect modifier would have been appropriate.** Note any additional comments: **None.**
What is the sample size? (specify total, cases/controls, exposed/unexposed, etc. as appropriate) N = 813 cases, N = 793 controls **Note only 810 cases completed questions on underarm hair removal and were included in analyses in this article**	Are sample size/power calculations provided? Is there sufficient statistical power for testing the stated hypotheses? **No power calculations provided; based on our own calculations using their results, they had 80% power to detect OR = 1.24 as statistically significant (type I error = 0.05; 30% prevalence of exclusive antiperspirant use among controls)** Note any additional comments: **None.**

Activities

Find a recently published observational study or randomized controlled trial on a topic of interest to you. You might consider using the article you read for the Activities from Chapter 7.

1. Complete Section 5 of the STAR template for this article to describe how the statistical analysis was conducted and evaluate the appropriateness of the statistical analysis approach.
2. Based on your answers to the questions in the STAR template, evaluate how the statistical analysis approach affects the internal validity of the study.
3. Think about other approaches to addressing confounding in the study. How might these other approaches serve to either strengthen or limit internal validity? Would these approaches be more or less feasible, given the study design and study population under study in the article?

References
1. Hart V, Reeves KW, Sturgeon SR, et al. The effect of change in body mass index on volumetric measures of mammographic density. *Cancer Epidemiol Biomark Prev.* 2015;24(11): 1724–1730. doi:10.1158/1055–9965.EPI-15–0330

2. Karwa S, Jahnke H, Brinson A, Shah N, Guille C, Henrich N. Association between Doula use on a digital health platform and birth outcomes. *Obstet Gynecol*. 2024;143(2): 175–183. doi:10.1097/AOG.0000000000005465

3. Frandsen CLB, Gottschau M, Nøhr B, et al. Polycystic ovary syndrome and endometrial cancer risk: Results from a nationwide cohort study. *Am J Epidemiol*. 2024;193(10): 1399–1406. doi:10.1093/aje/kwae061

4. Wu H, Reeves KW, Qian J, Sturgeon SR. Coffee, tea, and melanoma risk among post-menopausal women. *Eur J Cancer Prev*. 2015;24(4):347–352. doi:10.1097/CEJ. 0000000000000093

5. Kim S, Egerter S, Cubbin C, Takahashi ER, Braveman P. Potential implications of missing income data in population-based surveys: An example from a postpartum survey in California. *Public Health Rep*. 2007;122(6):753–763.

6. Little RJA, Rubin DB. *Statistical Analysis with Missing Data*. 3rd edition. Wiley; 2020.

7. FastStats. May 14, 2024. Accessed August 15, 2024. https://www.cdc.gov/nchs/fastats/ state-and-territorial-data.htm

8. Lash TL, VanderWeele TJ, Haneuse S, Rothman KJ, eds. *Modern Epidemiology*. 4th edition. Wolters Kluwer; 2021.

9. Savitz DA, Wellenius GA. *Interpreting Epidemiologic Evidence: Connecting Research to Applications*, 2nd ed. Oxford University Press; 2016.

10. Castaño-Vinyals G, Sadetzki S, Vermeulen R, et al. Wireless phone use in childhood and adolescence and neuroepithelial brain tumours: Results from the International MOBI-Kids Study. *Environ Int*. 2022;160. doi:10.1016/j.envint.2021.107069

11. Gammon MD, Neugut AI, Santella RM, et al. The Long Island Breast Cancer study project: Description of a multi-institutional collaboration to identify environmental risk factors for breast cancer. *Breast Cancer Res Treat*. 2002;74(3):235–254. doi:10.1023/A: 1016387020854

12. Missmer SA, Eliassen AH, Barbieri RL, Hankinson SE. Endogenous estrogen, androgen, and progesterone concentrations and breast cancer risk among postmenopausal women. *J Natl Cancer Inst*. 2004;96(24):1856–1865. doi:10.1093/jnci/djh336

13. Sacks FM, Svetkey LP, Vollmer WM, et al. Effects on blood pressure of reduced dietary sodium and the dietary approaches to stop hypertension (DASH) Diet. *N Engl J Med*. 2001;344(1):3–10. doi:10.1056/NEJM200101043440101

14. Crawford L, Reeves KW, Luisi N, Balasubramanian R, Sturgeon SR. Perineal powder use and risk of endometrial cancer in postmenopausal women. *Cancer Causes Control*. 2012;23(10):1673–1680. doi:10.1007/s10552-012-0046-3

15. Reeves KW, Okereke OI, Qian J, Tamimi RM, Eliassen AH, Hankinson SE. Depression, antidepressant use, and breast cancer risk in pre- and postmenopausal women: A prospective cohort study. *Cancer Epidemiol Biomark Prev*. 2018;27(3):306–314. doi:10.1158/1055–9965. EPI-17–0707

16. Endogenous Hormones Breast Cancer Collaborative Group. Body mass index, serum sex hormones, and breast cancer risk in postmenopausal women. *J Natl Cancer Inst*. 2003;95(16):1218–1226. doi:10.1093/jnci/djg022

17. Ursin G, Longnecker MP, Haile RW, Greenland S. A meta-analysis of body mass index and risk of premenopausal breast cancer. *Epidemiol*. 1995;6(2):137–141. doi:10.1097/ 00001648–199503000–00009

18. Mirick DK, Davis S, Thomas DB. Antiperspirant use and the risk of breast cancer. *J Natl Cancer Inst*. 2002;94(20):1578–1580. doi:10.1093/jnci/94.20.1578

CHAPTER 9

How do I write a critical analysis of an article?

Now that you know how to carefully identify and analyze every part of the study's methodology, you are (finally) ready to move on to the most interesting parts of the article: Results and Discussion. These are the sections where the authors will include multiple tables summarizing the results of their analysis and then provide their interpretation of what it all means in the context of their initial research question and other previous studies on the topic.

Your goal in writing a critical analysis paper is to share with your reader an objective and thorough evaluation of the article. (I recognize that your immediate goal may be to get an "A" on your assignment—but remember that the purpose of being assigned to write a critical analysis of an article is to give you practice developing this important skill.) Furthermore, you want to leave your reader with a clear understanding of what conclusions are appropriate to draw from the article—even if the conclusions *you* feel are appropriate are not the conclusions that the authors themselves make. A solid critical analysis will:

- include clear and accurate descriptions of the article's methods,
- correctly identify strengths and limitations relevant to each design feature,
- accurately evaluate the potential impact of these strengths and limitations on internal and external validity, and
- provide a clear and well-supported overall evaluation of the article.

In this chapter, you will learn how to write a critical analysis that is both thorough and concise.

What can I conclude from the article's results?

Before you begin writing your critical analysis, you need to have a clear understanding of what conclusions are appropriate to draw from the study described in the article. A good place to start is to identify what the authors report as their primary results.

DOI: 10.4324/9781003637899-10

Using Section 6 of the STAR template, you will take notes on the key findings of the article, including information on the direction and magnitude of measures of association.

You also will comment on how the authors assessed the stability of these results, which is often referred to as sensitivity analysis. For example, researchers often investigate if results are similar when reanalyzing the data using an alternative definition of the exposure or outcome, or after making modifications to key assumptions. Suppose, for instance, that a study sought to explore associations between illicit drug use and motor vehicle accidents. Ninety percent of the participants self-reported illicit drug use, while the exposure status of the remaining 10% was reported by a close contact of the participant (often referred to as reporting by "proxy"). The researchers may have been (rightly) concerned about bias resulting from exposure misclassification from the proxy reports. After their initial analysis, it would be useful to conduct additional analyses to examine whether the primary results were overly influenced by the proxy responses. In this next set of analyses, the researchers might exclude participants whose exposure was reported by a proxy and reanalyze the data. They would then evaluate the extent to which the findings from these additional analyses are similar to those of the initial analysis. The idea is that if the proxy responses were unbiased, then the direction and magnitude of the effect estimate should be similar when they are excluded. Note that I did not say statistical significance because excluding a subset of participants (here, the 10% with exposure reported by a proxy) will decrease the sample size, the statistical power will be decreased also. In this type of sensitivity analysis, statistical significance is less important than the consistency (or inconsistency) with the initial findings.

The STAR template also asks you to record the conclusions that the authors make. Here, I find that using a direct quotation can be helpful, as the exact tone and wording are often important in the statement of conclusions (just don't forget to use quotation marks to indicate that you are taking the authors' words verbatim). On the right-hand side in Section 6, you will note whether these conclusions are appropriate given the article's reported results, explaining why or why not. Importantly, if you do not feel that the authors' conclusions are justified, describe what conclusions *you* feel are appropriate to draw from the article. For example, if the authors describe a strong association between exposure and outcome and cite an OR of 2.5 (95% CI 0.8–3.4), you would be correct in noting that the study *suggests* a positive association, but that the result was not statistically significant (Table 9.1).

STAR in action: examining the results and conclusions in Mirick et al.

Mirick et al.[1] conclude that there is no association between antiperspirant/deodorant use and breast cancer risk. For example, neither regular use of antiperspirants (OR 0.9, 95% CI 0.7–1.1) nor regular use of deodorants (OR 1.2, 95% 0.9–1.5) was statistically significantly associated with breast cancer risk. Similar findings were observed when exclusive use of each product or use within 1 hr of shaving was assessed. The authors' conclusions are appropriate based on the results of their statistical analysis. This was the first epidemiologic assessment of whether antiperspirant/deodorant use affects breast cancer risk, and the results do not support a causal association.

Table 9.1 Completed STAR template section 6: "Results and Conclusions" for Mirick et al. (2002)[1]

6. *Results and conclusions*

What was the major result of the study? Include information on direction and magnitude of association for the most important finding. [e.g., Give the actual OR and confidence interval, and also interpret the findings in words. Be sure to mention the comparison category in your text (e.g., compared to individuals who did not drink alcohol)

There is no association between deodorant/antiperspirant use and breast cancer risk.

Adjusted ORs as reported in Table 1:

Antiperspirant use exclusively: OR 0.8, 95% CI 0.6–1.0

Antiperspirant use regularly: OR 0.9, 95% CI 0.7–1.1

Antiperspirant use within 1 hr of shaving: OR 0.9, 95% CI 0.7–1.1

Deodorant use exclusively: OR 1.1, 95% CI 0.9–1.4

Deodorant use regularly: OR 1.2, 95% CI 0.9–1.5

Deodorant use within 1 hr of shaving: OR 1.2, 95% CI 0.9–1.5

Was the stability of the result assessed (i.e., did the authors report subgroup and/or stratified analyses, explore alternative exposure and/or outcome definitions, etc.?) If so, describe the analyses and their results.

Yes, authors considered multiple approaches for measuring exposure (i.e., exclusive use, regular use, use within 1 hr of shaving); results are generally consistent in showing no association between these exposures and breast cancer.

What conclusions do the authors make?
The authors conclude that there is no evidence of an association between antiperspirant or deodorant use and breast cancer risk.

Are these conclusions justified, given the results? Why or why not? If not, what conclusions do you feel are appropriate?
Yes, these conclusions are accurate given the null findings (i.e., ORs close to 1 and 95% CIs including 1).

How do these findings compare to those of prior studies? What factors might account for any differences noted?
The authors state that this is the first epidemiologic study to evaluate this research question; thus, there is not a comparison made to prior epidemiologic research.

Note any additional comments:
None.

How do I come up with an overall assessment of the article?

At this point, you have finished reading the article. You have carefully identified and analyzed every aspect of the study, from its overall design, to the criteria used to select the study population, to how the exposure and outcome were measured, and finally, to how the data were analyzed. You have identified their primary results and drawn our own conclusions. Now, all you need to do is pull it all together. Sounds easy, right?

If you continue utilizing the STAR template, arriving at an overall assessment (Section 7) actually isn't too hard. First, you will think through all the various strengths and limitations you have identified as you read the article and noted in Sections 1–6. Here, you want to focus on just the *most important* strengths and limitations. It's perfectly fine to copy and paste what you wrote about those strengths and limitations in earlier sections of the STAR template. Your goal in Section 7 is to pull together the key information that forms our overall assessment of the article, which also will make it easier when you write your critical analysis. For each of the important strengths and limitations you note, describe the methodology that led to the strength or limitation, how it affects internal and external validity, and whether its potential effect on the study's results is minor, moderate, or major.

Once you've done that, you can use that information to characterize the overall quality of the study and then write a brief summary of the article. This brief summary will be very helpful as a starting point for your critical analysis (and also helpful if you need to quickly remember your thoughts on this article in the future). While I probably don't need to tell you how to write a brief summary, you are likely wondering how to judge the quality of an article. Let's tackle that question next, before moving on to writing the critical analysis itself.

How do I judge the quality of the article?

First, let's establish what the "quality" of the article means. You could think about quality in several ways: was the article well-written? Was it published in a reputable peer-reviewed journal? *When critically analyzing a scientific article, though, your primary goal is to assess the extent to which the article's findings are internally valid.* When you describe the "quality" of the article, this is essentially shorthand for describing its internal validity.

Evaluating the quality of individual articles is an important part of establishing the level of confidence in the literature addressing the research question. It is also important to note, though, that judging the quality of an individual article is separate from judging the quality of the overall evidence on a given topic. The latter is extremely important when making clinical recommendations and setting policy. In these cases, it is more helpful to think about the validity of the evidence rather than describing this as quality.[2]

So, how do you measure the quality of an article? Many different approaches have been developed, most of which utilize a scoring system in an attempt to create an objective measurement. For example, the non-profit Cochrane organization facilitated the development of "Risk of Bias" tools for experimental and observational studies by large groups of scientific experts.[3]

I won't advocate for a particular scoring system. Descriptors of quality can be helpful to readers, but any system will have room for error and improvement. In fact, while it would be wonderful to have a quantitative and wholly objective way to rate article quality, this just is not possible. Quality depends on too many factors. And too many of those factors are subject to your own interpretation and comfort level.

Imagine a prospective cohort study that measured antidepressant use as its primary exposure using a self-administered questionnaire. You and I agree that there are important limitations to this approach, mainly the potential for non-differential misclassification, given inaccuracies in how participants report their prior and current use of these medications. But, we could easily disagree on the relative importance of this limitation; I might place it in the "minor issue" bucket, while you might instead put it in the "moderate issue" bucket. I could point to people being generally good at reporting their medications, while you could point to there being social stigma around antidepressants, and thus, people might be likely to underreport their use. In the end, we might have to agree to disagree.

Ultimately, the judgment of article quality is somewhat subjective. This is why I suggest that you use the descriptors "excellent," "good," and "poor" to rate the article's quality (Table 9.2). These are the options you will find in Section 7 of the STAR template. In my experience, these three descriptors provide sufficient information. More options of quality categories generally lead to more time spent debating between them (e.g., whether an article is "fair" or "good" or "very good"), when the differences across those categories probably aren't big enough to be useful.

An "excellent" article would have many major strengths and any limitations would minimally impact internal validity; a "poor" article would be just the opposite. We each have our own internal definitions of what makes an article "excellent" versus "good" versus "poor." While you and I might disagree on which descriptor we choose between neighboring categories (e.g., excellent vs good), we can typically agree on the extremes (i.e., we both agree that the excellent/good article is definitely not poor).

Whatever quality rating you choose, the descriptor should be consistent with the overall balance of strengths and limitations that you have identified. These strengths and limitations were identified and discussed in relation to their impact on internal validity, and the description of an article's quality is essentially shorthand for internal validity. So, it makes sense that an "excellent" article would have many strengths (and few limitations), while a "poor" article would have many limitations (and few strengths).

At this point you might be thinking, "if we can't come up with an objective way to measure article quality, why even bother?" This is a valid point. My view, however, is that labeling the quality of an article is helpful, both to you and to your reader. The label helps to organize your thoughts as you write the critical analysis, setting the tone

Table 9.2 Describing the article's "quality" is essentially a shorthand for its internal validity and can be helpful in organizing your thoughts and setting the tone for writing your critical analysis

	Article quality		
	Poor	*Good*	*Excellent*
Strengths	Few or none	Some or many	Many
Limitations	Many	Some or many	Few or none
Internal validity	Low	Moderate	High

for how you present the article to your readers. And, using a word like "poor" versus "excellent" to describe the article early on lets your readers know what to expect and how to judge the validity of the article's conclusions. Additionally, when you begin to synthesize evidence across multiple studies, identifying those studies that are of better quality (really, higher internal validity) versus those that are of poorer quality (really, lower internal validity) will help you to weigh the evidence and come up with an overall conclusion about what the literature is telling you.

One additional important reminder before you write the critical analysis itself: it's completely acceptable to say a study is good (or even excellent) if this indeed is the case. I find that students have a tendency to say all studies are of poor quality, even if they have listed many strengths and relatively few limitations. Maybe it's the word "critical" that makes them think that they have to say the article is bad. Students always seem surprised when I assign them to critically analyze a study that, in my view, is excellent. It seems like a trick. The truth is that while no study is perfect, many studies really are quite good (even excellent). While it is important to acknowledge limitations and how they impact internal validity, it also is important to communicate when these limitations are outweighed by strengths, resulting in a study with high internal validity from which we can draw important conclusions (Table 9.3).

Table 9.3 Completed STAR template section 7: "Overall Assessment" for Mirick et al. (2002)[1]

---

7. *Overall assessment*

What are the most important strengths of the study? For each, describe in detail why this is an important strength and how it affects internal and/or external validity. Is the potential effect of the strength on the results minor, moderate or major?

- Outcome assessment: cancer diagnoses ascertained via cancer registry minimize differential and non-differential misclassification of outcome; a major impact on internal validity
  - Minimal chance of selection bias: cases and controls were selected from same source population using well-defined and similar criteria, cases and controls have similar and high response rates; a major impact on internal validity
  - Adjustment for confounders: multivariable regression adjusted for many potential confounders, although residual confounding remains possible; a major impact on internal validity

---

What are the most important limitations of the study? For each, describe in detail why this is an important limitation and how it affects internal and/or external validity? Is the potential effect of the limitation on the results minor, moderate, or major?

- Exposure assessment: major potential for non-differential misclassification of exposure due to general difficulty in remembering these prior exposures, also moderate potential for differential misclassification of exposure due to recall bias and/or interviewer bias; non-differential misclassification would tend to bias associations toward the null, while the differential misclassification could bias observed associations away from the null; given the null findings observed, it is possible that they could be the result of non-differential misclassification

---

(Continued)

Table 9.3 *(Continued)*

7. Overall assessment

- ■ Retrospective case-control design lacks temporality and relates directly to the exposure assessment issues noted above
- ■ Lack of racial/ethnic diversity means that it is reasonable to question whether these findings apply to non-White individuals; while the biologic mechanism would not differ, different patterns of use in other racial/ethnic groups (including frequency and type) might show associations with breast cancer risk that were not observable given the exposure range in the White study population

How would you characterize the overall quality of the study?

☐ Poor **X Good** ☐ Excellent

Justify your choice.
While the study has important limitations, there are many strengths that enhance internal validity.

Write a <u>brief</u> summary of the article, describing the key methodologic elements, strengths, limitations, and the conclusions that are most appropriate given the article's findings and your assessment of internal validity:
In this case-control study of 810 incident breast cancer cases and 793 controls, there was no statistically significant association observed between various measures of antiperspirant and deodorant use and breast cancer risk (e.g., OR 0.9, 95% CI 0.7–1.1 for ever vs never regular use of antiperspirants). Breast cancer cases were identified through a population-based cancer registry in Washington State, with controls identified from this same geographic area and frequency-matched to cases in 5-year age groups. The rigorous methods used to identify cases minimize potential for outcome misclassification, thus substantially enhancing the study's internal validity. Additionally, cases and controls were enrolled based on similar eligibility criteria, with high response rates for both cases (78%) and controls (75%), thus minimizing concerns of selection bias. However, the retrospective case-control design lacks appropriate temporality for the exposure-outcome relationship. This design also raises concerns around the exposure assessment, as prior use of antiperspirants and deodorants might be difficult to remember and recall and also could differ between cases and controls. Both differential and non-differential misclassification of exposure is possible and likely had at least a moderate effect on the study findings. The study used multivariable logistic regression to estimate adjusted odds ratios and 95% confidence intervals, reducing the potential for confounding to affect the results. Overall, this is a good quality study with results that are judged to be internally valid. However, the external validity is somewhat questionable as only White participants were included. While biologic mechanisms linking antiperspirants/deodorants to breast cancer risk are unlikely to vary by race/ethnicity, differing exposure patterns may mean that an association could be observed if other racial/ethnic groups have higher exposures and there is a threshold of exposure at which breast cancer risk is impacted.

STAR in action: formulating an overall assessment of Mirick et al.

This population-based case-control study[1] has numerous strengths that enhance its internal validity. Among them, the outcome assessment, through the state cancer registry, minimizes the potential for both non-differential and differential misclassification of outcomes. Also, because cases and controls were selected from the same source population using well-defined and similar criteria, the potential for selection bias is low. Further, the high response rates among both cases and controls reduce the likelihood of selection bias. The results are further strengthened by thorough adjustment for confounders using multivariable logistic regression.

However, a few limitations that impact internal validity must be noted. First, the exposure assessment, via interviewer-administered questionnaires, has a major potential for non-differential misclassification of exposure. The exposure of interest, antiperspirant and/or deodorant use prior to diagnosis, may be difficult for participants to remember and report accurately, which would tend to bias results toward finding no association. The results indicated no association between use of antiperspirants and/or deodorants, potentially resulting from non-differential misclassification. However, there is also a potential for differential misclassification, if cases and controls differ in their accuracy of reporting due to either recall bias and/or interviewer bias. Both the non-differential and the differential misclassification of exposure relate directly to the retrospective study design, which calls into question the temporality of the exposure–outcome relationship. Finally, another important limitation is the lack of racial/ethnic diversity of the study population. Because only White participants were included and because patterns of exposure differ across races/ethnicities, it is reasonable to question whether the results observed within this study population would be applicable to racially/ethnically diverse populations.

Overall, this study is judged to have good internal validity and supports the conclusion that antiperspirants/deodorants are not associated with breast cancer risk. Due to the noted limitations, especially the lack of racial/ethnic diversity, future studies evaluating the research question in racially/ethnically diverse study populations with a prospective study design are warranted.

How do I turn my notes from the STAR template into text?

As I've said many times by now, writing a clear and thoughtful critical analysis of a scientific journal article is a key skill for epidemiologists. An effective critical analysis will evaluate the key features of the study—i.e., the study design, study population, exposure assessment, outcome assessment, statistical approaches, and other methods—in relation to how they affect the internal and external validity of the study. It is equally important to identify the features that are strengths of the study as it is to identify those that are limitations. You should cite evidence from the article to support any statements you make and explain why the feature is a strength or limitation.

A well-written critical analysis of an epidemiologic article tends to be around 6–8 double-spaced pages. You might not think this is long enough to include all the elements of the study and clearly explain your critical analysis. Writing concisely is difficult, but it is also an important skill for epidemiologists. In my experience, this length is sufficient for covering the article thoroughly (note: your professors might disagree—follow whatever length requirements they give you. After all, they are the ones assigning your grade!). In the "real world" (e.g., in writing a grant), you often will be reducing your critical analysis of an entire article to a sentence or two. So, it is important to learn how to write concisely now.

Box 9.1

Tips for overcoming writer's block

We've all been there: staring at a blank page or screen, amazing thoughts swirling in our heads, and a complete inability to write any of them down. Writer's block can be incredibly frustrating, and getting unstuck often feels impossible. While I am not a professional writing coach, I have spent a lot of time writing myself and advising students on their writing. Here are some approaches to getting unstuck that have worked for me (and my students) over the years:

- **Accept writer's block as part of the process.** Most writers experience writer's block. Accepting that it will happen to you, too, makes it a bit less frustrating. Build time into your writing schedule to allow yourself to get unstuck.
- **Create an outline.** This doesn't need to be a perfect outline using parallel structure and all the levels of headings you learned in high school. Start with the outline or assignment description given to you. Use bullet points and incomplete, poorly written sentences just to get your ideas out. Then, move them around to get them into a coherent order. The outline is just for you, so don't worry about spelling words correctly or writing beautiful prose. Those things can come later. The important first step is just to get your ideas out onto the page. Revising tends to be far easier than creating.
- **View the first draft as one giant mistake.** I would bet that less than 50% of what I write in my first draft actually makes it into my final product, whether I am writing a grant application, a manuscript, or even this book. Don't expect your first draft to be perfect—it won't come even close. Your goal is just to get your ideas out, and then you can fine-tune the writing from there.
- **Set a timer.** The Pomodoro[4] is a popular model. Set a timer for 25 minutes, get rid of distractions (email, phones, other people…) and start writing. Then, set another timer for 5 minutes and take a break. Somehow, knowing you only have to write for 25 minutes (and also that you will get to do something you enjoy after that) makes it feel much more doable. Use whatever time periods work best for you. I often find that when my timer goes off, I am in the zone and just keep on writing.
- **Record yourself.** I wish I had a dollar for every time a student sat in my office saying they weren't sure how to write something, then proceeded to give me a very clear and detailed explanation of exactly what they wanted to say. "Write that!" I always tell them. When we speak, we tend not to edit ourselves and perseverate over word choices and grammatical structure—the ideas just flow. Take advantage of this fact and record yourself explaining to someone else (even a pet will do) what it is you want to say. Then, transcribe what you've said.
- **Cover up your screen.** I find that when I am looking at my screen, I am trying to edit at the same time I am trying to write. Instead of focusing on the ideas, I end up focusing too much on word choice and writing clarity. Somehow, if I don't look at the screen, I stop doing this. My mind is free to just let the ideas come out through my fingers, and I am not paying any attention to whether I have spelled that last word correctly or if I need a comma somewhere. You could close your eyes, put a piece of paper in front of your screen, or even force yourself to watch your fingers as

they type. Anything to allow your brain to separate the initial writing process from the editing process.

■ **Use placeholders.** I very often find that I can get 90% of the sentence written, but then I get stuck on a particular word that I've used too much or isn't quite right, or an idea that I need to explain better or research further. This can really get me stuck and bring my writing process to a screeching halt. Using placeholders to indicate something you need to come back to later can help restore that flow. This could be as simple as writing XXX in a spot that needs something more, highlighting text that you know will need revision, or writing a note to yourself in brackets. Your future self can deal with the issue later, while your present self can keep writing.

■ **Join a writing group.** Nothing is more motivating than telling a group of friends (or, better yet, strangers) what your goals are. Writing accountability groups have gained popularity within academia. While the exact structure may vary, participation generally involves meeting at regularly scheduled times, telling each other your writing goals for that session, and then getting to work. At the end of the session, everyone checks in again and says whether or not they accomplished their goal, and then sets a writing goal to accomplish on their own before the next meeting. Accountability without judgment can be amazingly helpful. And, having set times on your schedule to write also ensures you give yourself time to focus on the task.

■ **Take a break.** Go outside. Take a walk. Talk to a friend. Get a snack. Anything that gets you away from staring at your screen and thinking about how you just can't seem to write. Spending 15 minutes being frustrated in front of your computer isn't going to suddenly make the words flow. But using those same 15 minutes to take a break to clear your head might (and usually does). Even better, switch your environment when you get back to writing—sometimes a new space helps you get a fresh start.

Getting started with writing can be challenging, to say the least (see Box 9.1 for some ideas for getting past writer's block). If you have taken careful notes using the STAR template, though, you will find the process of writing your critical analysis to be far easier. The critical analysis itself should follow the general structure described in Table 9.4, which you might notice is quite similar to the structure of the STAR template. In your written critical analysis, though, you should add an introductory paragraph to give an overview of the article. This paragraph reports the key details of the study, which you recorded on the lefthand side of your STAR template. Keep the introductory paragraph strictly a description of the methodology, without commenting on strengths and limitations or how they impact validity—that will come in the following sections. Here, let me also remind you to be careful to paraphrase and not copy the language verbatim from the article (unless you use quotation marks and an appropriate citation).

Next, use the notes from the righthand side of the STAR template to write a thoughtful critical analysis of each of the major aspects of the study methodology. It is helpful to use the same headings on the STAR template in your written critical analysis, that is, Study Population, Exposure Assessment, Outcome Assessment, and Statistical Analysis. Now is your opportunity to bring in your interpretation of the study.

Table 9.4 General outline for a written article critical analysis

A. Overview of study (~1 paragraph)

The goal of this paragraph is to describe the key methodologic features of the article, without commentary or analysis. Provide a concise description of the:

- Purpose/background context
- Study design
- Study participants
- Exposure of interest and how its measured
- Outcome of interest and how its measured
- Statistical analysis
- Primary results

B. Study population (~1–2 paragraphs)
C. Exposure assessment (~1–2 paragraphs)
D. Outcome assessment (~1–2 paragraphs)
E. Statistical analysis (~1–2 paragraphs)

In each of the above sections (B–E), specifically discuss how the relevant methods are either strengths or limitations and impact internal and external validity, identifying issues as minimal, moderate, or major impact. Comment on key methodologic issues as appropriate, e.g., selection bias, differential misclassification, non-differential misclassification, confounding, effect modification, and chance.

F. Overall assessment (~1–3 paragraphs)

Synthesize your comments from the above sections (B–E), highlighting the most important strengths and limitations to support your overall evaluation of the article and statement of what you feel can be concluded from the research. Address the following questions/items:

- How would you characterize the overall quality of the study? Explain your choice.
- What are the *most important* strengths of the study? Describe why these are strengths and how they affect internal and/or external validity.
- What are the *most important* limitations of the study? Describe why these are limitations and how they affect internal and/or external validity.
- Based on your responses to the above questions, what conclusions are appropriate from the article? Are the results generalizable?
- How do the article's results compare to other studies on the same topic and/or on related topics?

G. References

Provide a complete citation for the article that you are critically analyzing, as well as any other literature you refer to within your paper.

You should specifically discuss how the relevant methods are either strengths or limitations and impact internal and external validity, identifying issues as having a minimal, moderate, or major impact. Comment on key methodologic issues as appropriate (e.g., selection bias, differential misclassification, non-differential misclassification, confounding, effect modification, and chance). As you write your critical analysis, focus on the most important strengths and limitations; you already identified these in Section 7 of the STAR template. Your critical analysis should focus mainly on the "major" and "moderate" internal validity buckets, providing a thorough explanation of why each feature is a strength (or limitation) and how it affects internal validity.

Finally, you will write a concluding section providing your overall assessment of the article (referring to the notes you made in Section 7 of the STAR template). You will also need to put the study's results into context with other published literature on the topic. Well-written articles will do this as part of the Discussion section. But recognize that an author's write up might be a bit slanted, downplaying their own weaknesses while playing up those of others. Poorly written articles might ignore studies whose findings contradict their own. Excellent articles will acknowledge and fully discuss their own limitations, and how they impact internal validity, and how these compare to those of other studies. In other words, a careful reading of the Discussion section is a good starting point, but you'll need to do more than just that. Sometimes, this will even mean that you need to do your own search of the literature to find similar articles and then read and critically analyze those articles, too. When writing a critical analysis of a single article, you likely won't need to write an extended discussion of how the study fits into the broader literature on the topic, but you should spend at least a paragraph situating the study within the literature. Synthesizing results from multiple studies on a single topic is itself an important skill, which we will tackle in Chapter 10. A more thorough Discussion section will be needed for a systematic literature review, which we will cover in Chapter 11.

How do I effectively communicate my critical analysis in writing?

I tend to think of writing as making an argument, not in the "I'm mad" sense, but in the "I want to convince you to think the way I do" sense. And the best way to convince your reader of your point of view is to be clear and concise and to cite evidence to back up your statements. Scientific writing tends to be short and to the point—now is not the time to use flowery language and long, complex sentences. Concise writing is especially important as you transition to writing grant applications or journal articles, both of which will have very strict page or word count limitations. My general rule of thumb is that if a sentence covers more than two typed lines, it needs to be made into (at least) two shorter sentences. Also, plain language is always better than complicated language. Your audience, whether it is your professor grading dozens of critical analyses or a reviewer reading dozens of grants, will appreciate that you've made their job easier by writing clearly.

Throughout your critical analysis, you will be building your argument for how you think the reader should view the article and its conclusions. This argument should be logical and support your evaluation of the article's quality. For example, if your analysis of the various study design elements consistently points out more strengths than limitations, your final assessment of the article's quality should fall into the good or excellent range. It would be surprising to your reader if you concluded that the article was of poor quality if you only ever pointed out minor limitations.

As you build your case, use evidence from the article to support your analysis. If you identify a design feature as a strength, explain why it enhances the study's validity. Likewise, if you identify a design feature as a limitation, explain how it creates an opportunity for bias or error. For example, if you state that the external validity is limited, support this by showing how the study population lacks representativeness on key features. Or, if you note that recall bias affected the exposure assessment, explain exactly how this occurred and what impact it is likely to have on the study's results.

Make sure that your critical analysis covers all aspects of the study. Follow the critical analysis outline provided in Table 9.4 (which matches the STAR template) so that you don't inadvertently skip one of the key methodologic elements. This doesn't mean that each element will get equal real estate in your critical analysis. If the study's population is relatively straightforward and without important limitations, you may be able to thoroughly cover this topic in a brief paragraph. On the other hand, if the outcome assessment is problematic and has substantial opportunities for bias and error, you will need to thoroughly cover these issues in a longer paragraph (or more). It may be helpful to add sub-sections to your critical analysis depending on the nature of the article and the extent of the strengths and limitations (e.g., if the article focuses on multiple exposures, you may wish to have sub-sections devoted to each one within your section on exposure assessment).

As you write, take care to avoid plagiarism. I know I have said this already, but it is worth repeating because it is so important. You should paraphrase as much as possible, saving direct quotations for only the very key statements the authors make and where their voice is truly needed (such as quoting their statement of conclusions). Hopefully, you have heeded my earlier advice as you have been completing the STAR template and have paraphrased as you took notes or at least used quotation marks to indicate where your notes are verbatim from the article. In my experience, most cases of plagiarism among students are unintentional and arise from sloppy notetaking and/or insufficient paraphrasing. But, unintentional plagiarism is still plagiarism.

Can you give me an example of a well-written critical analysis?

Absolutely! Throughout this textbook, I have used the STAR template to help critically analyze the article by Mirick et al.[1] Appendix B includes a full-length written critical analysis of this article, based on the notes I recorded in the STAR template. You will note that this critical analysis adheres to the outline provided in Table 9.4 (although, it is on the short side, given that the original article was published as a "brief communication"). As you read the critical analysis included in Appendix B, pay attention to the concise writing style. I hope you also will note that the critical analysis goes beyond simply naming a strength or limitation and also includes an explanation of *why* the methodologic component serves to increase or decrease the study's internal and/or external validity.

Activities

Find a recently published observational study or randomized controlled trial on a topic of interest to you. You might consider using the article you read for the Activities from Chapter 8.

1. Complete Section 6 of the STAR template for this article to identify and evaluate the article's results and conclusions.
2. Complete Section 7 of the STAR template to identify the most important strengths and limitations of the article and form an overall assessment.
3. Using your notes from the STAR template and following the outline provided in Table 9.4, write a critical analysis of the article.

References

1. Mirick DK, Davis S, Thomas DB. Antiperspirant use and the risk of breast cancer. *J Natl Cancer Inst*. 2002;94(20):1578–1580. doi:10.1093/jnci/94.20.1578
2. Page MJ, McKenzie JE, Bossuyt PM, et al. The PRISMA 2020 statement: An updated guideline for reporting systematic reviews. *BMJ*. 2021;372:n71. doi:10.1136/bmj.n71
3. Risk of Bias 2 (RoB 2) Tool | Cochrane Methods. Accessed June 25, 2024. https://methods.cochrane.org/risk-bias-2
4. Pomodoro® Technique - Time Management Method. Accessed June 24, 2024. https://www.pomodorotechnique.com

CHAPTER 10

How do I synthesize evidence across studies?

As I noted in the Introduction to this textbook, a single study is never definitive. By now, it should be obvious to you why this is true: epidemiologic studies are all subject to limitations, and there is no such thing as a "perfect" study.

Because epidemiologists study humans, not lab rats, it is basically impossible to "replicate" an epidemiologic study. Even if you were to use the same recruitment procedures, ask the same questions, and measure the same outcomes, you would still be studying different people at different times. This means that studies in human populations have far more to contend with than just random error. You need to consider the impact of all the different biases and threats to validity within each individual study, and you must then consider the results of multiple studies on a given topic together to arrive at an overall conclusion. But, how do you actually do that?

Most journal articles will include a comparison of their findings to previous literature in the Discussion section and will make some overall statements about what the study adds to the scientific understanding of the topic at hand. While consistency across studies is an important part of demonstrating causality, there are many reasons why two different studies of the same exposure-outcome relationship could produce dissimilar results (yet both could have high internal validity).

In this chapter you will learn how to compare and contrast multiple epidemiologic studies, weighing the strengths and limitations of each one to reach an overall conclusion. This is itself an important skill. Healthcare providers will need to synthesize results across studies to make an evidence-based decision about treatment approaches, and scientists will need to synthesize findings across studies to identify gaps in the literature or to convince funding agencies to support their work.

As you will see, this is more complicated than simply tallying the number of studies on a given topic that found a positive/negative/null result and then using the highest tally to form your conclusion. You need to consider the quality of the various studies as well as how differences in their findings may (or may not) be explained by differences in methodology. Your ultimate goal is to provide a thoughtful and

DOI: 10.4324/9781003637899-11

objective evaluation of the literature as a whole and to put the findings of each article into context with one another.

Why can't I just count the number of studies that found a positive (or negative, or null) result?

If only it were as straightforward as counting, this would be a very short chapter indeed. Unfortunately, simply counting the number of studies that found a certain result is essentially useless. I know what you're thinking: isn't consistency important? Technically, yes. But what if the consistent results come from studies that all have poor internal validity? It is possible that consistent results could reflect a consistent set of limitations and thus still be wrong!

Additionally, focusing only on the direction of the reported association overlooks other important considerations, namely its magnitude and its precision. As we have discussed, statistical power plays an important role in drawing conclusions from studies. Imagine an underpowered study that reports a non-statistically significant (e.g., $p = 0.09$) positive association. If we include this study in our tally of "null" reports, we would be excluding evidence of a potential positive association that might be apparent with higher statistical power. Furthermore, we should also consider the strength of the reported association. A statistically significant OR = 1.5 from a highly valid study is more compelling, for example, than a statistically significant OR = 5.0 from another, less valid, study. If we only count the number of studies with positive, statistically significant results, we overlook the differences in the strength of the association and the opportunity to consider why that might be.

Why would different studies reach different conclusions?

Differences in study results often relate to differences in methodology across the studies (Figure 10.1). Instead of simply tallying the *number* of positive/negative/null results, you need to evaluate each study independently in terms of its internal and external validity. As you consider the findings of multiple studies on your topic of interest, you will want to put more weight on those derived from high-quality studies, and less weight on those from studies of lesser quality. (If you haven't already, read the section in Chapter 9 on how to assess the quality of scientific articles.)

High-quality studies could still arrive at different conclusions. Different studies in different populations using a different approach to measurement of exposure and/ or outcome can each be valid *and* can have different results. And they can each be right! Even if a set of studies considers the same exposure-outcome association and measures the exposure and outcome in the same way, the *participants* in those studies are different. As a result, the range of exposure and other important confounding or effect-modifying variables could be different, too. Again, people are not like lab rats whose genetics, environment, and exposures you can carefully control. It is critical that you consider each component of the study methodology as you seek to understand what, at first glance, appear to be "inconsistencies" across study results.

Imagine that three high-quality studies of a population with low exposure to perfluoroalkyl substances (PFAS) reported no association between PFAS and child neurological development, while a fourth study that included a broader (and higher) range

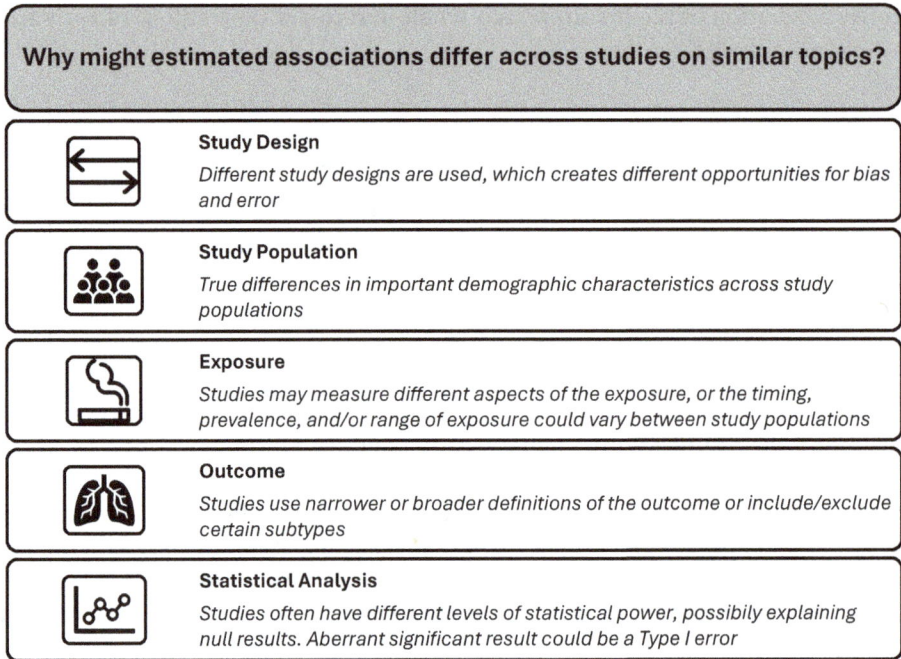

Why might estimated associations differ across studies on similar topics?

Study Design
Different study designs are used, which creates different opportunities for bias and error

Study Population
True differences in important demographic characteristics across study populations

Exposure
Studies may measure different aspects of the exposure, or the timing, prevalence, and/or range of exposure could vary between study populations

Outcome
Studies use narrower or broader definitions of the outcome or include/exclude certain subtypes

Statistical Analysis
Studies often have different levels of statistical power, possibily explaining null results. Aberrant significant result could be a Type I error

Figure 10.1 Epidemiologic studies can never be exactly replicated, and even high-quality studies of similar exposure-outcome relationships may generate different results.

of PFAS exposure found a strong, positive association between PFAS and neurological developmental delays in children. Would you simply conclude that, because three is more than one, there is no association? No. You would want to consider that all four studies could have high internal validity, but that perhaps the association between PFAS and neurological development is only apparent at higher exposure levels.

Another possibility is that differences across studies could reflect true differences across populations (in other words, effect modification). Imagine a high-quality study of obesity and breast cancer in premenopausal women that reports a negative association, while a similarly high-quality study of obesity and breast cancer in postmenopausal women reports a positive association. As discussed in Chapter 8, menopausal status *modifies* the effect of obesity on breast cancer. Studies that only (or primarily) include premenopausal women compared to those that only (or primarily) include postmenopausal women will arrive at different results due to true effect modification reflecting differing physiologic mechanisms between pre- and postmenopausal women. In other words, you are comparing the proverbial apples to oranges.

Lack of external validity also could be to blame for differences across studies. This might especially be true if the exposure-outcome relationship is affected by important social and/or socioeconomic differences (i.e., if there is effect modification by these factors). In such cases, apparent differences in the exposure–outcome relationship across studies could actually be due to important differences in the socioeconomic and/or social situations of the participants in each study, which do not confound the results of the individual studies since they represent "restricted" samples (i.e., participants are of similar socioeconomic status, for example), but which does explain the differences across studies. For example, associations between race/ethnicity and heart attack mortality might differ substantially across studies conducted in populations with and without access to high-quality emergency medical care.

Sometimes, it turns out that the exposure under study is not actually the same across the various studies. For example, you might have found five studies evaluating whether social media use is a risk factor for depression. Based on their abstracts, these studies seem to all be studying the same exposure and the same outcome. But when you read the Methods section, you might find that they all use different definitions and measurements of social media use. Some only measure use within the past year, while others define use as ever versus never. Some only ask about certain apps, while others leave "social media" open to the participants' interpretation of what qualifies as social media. In reality, these studies are all measuring different aspects of social media. The measured exposure is not actually the same, although the studies are all trying to measure the same construct. To the extent that these different aspects have a different impact on the outcome, you could expect to see inconsistency across the studies.

And what about that outcome? Imagine that some studies are measuring depressive symptoms while others are measuring a prior or current diagnosis, and still others are measuring severe depression requiring hospitalization. Again, these might first appear to all be studies on "depression," but in reality, they are measuring different aspects or subtypes of depression. Taking that one step further, you might also expect that social media would have a different association with depressive symptoms than it does with severe depression requiring hospitalization.

A final consideration is the role of random error and statistical power. You need to consider that a well-powered study could find a statistically significant association (e.g., RR 1.4, 95% CI 1.1–1.8), while a poorly powered study might find a similar magnitude and direction of association, but one that is not statistically significant (e.g., RR 1.4, 95% CI 0.8–1.6). So, what might first appear to be an inconsistency, could actually be thought of as consistent if you instead focus on the direction and magnitude of association and consider the implications of the lack of statistical power in the latter study. Additionally, random variation will impact all studies, so you should never expect to find *exactly* the same results in one study as you do in another (e.g., the exact same OR and 95% confidence interval). You should expect random variation to occur across studies (and, in fact, seeing results that are identical across studies should cause you to raise your eyebrows and investigate a bit further...). You also need to keep in mind that if you use a Type I error rate of 0.05, then one out of every twenty statistical tests will be making a Type I error (i.e., rejecting the null hypothesis when the null hypothesis is true). As a result, you shouldn't put too much stock in the one statistically significant result among a sea of otherwise null findings; it could be that this result is an artifact of statistical testing and random error.

How can I organize information from multiple studies on a similar topic?

Keeping track of the various methodologic details for each study can be challenging, especially if you have more than two or three studies to compare and contrast. I find it helpful to create a table to help organize the relevant information from multiple studies. Such a table should include columns for each of the key methodologic aspects: study design, population (including sample size), exposure definition and measurement, outcome definition and measurement, primary results, key strengths, and key limitations (Table 10.1).

Table 10.1 Example of a table summarizing key information for a hypothetical set of studies evaluating a similar research question (i.e., exposure–outcome relationship)

Author (year) study design	Study population	BMI at age 50 (exposure)	Dementia (outcome)	Main result BMI ≥30 kg/m² vs <30 kg/m²	Key strengths	Key limitations	Quality
Author A (2015) **Case-control**	100 cases from local hospital, and 100 controls from university faculty/staff in a neighboring state	Self-reported	Self-reported	OR = 5.0 (95% CI 0.8–9.5)	■ None noted	■ Retrospective design ■ High potential for selection bias given cases and controls recruited from different source populations ■ High potential for recall bias (differential misclassification of exposure) ■ Low statistical power	Poor
Author B (2019) **Prospective cohort**	1000 older adults recruited from senior center, with 35% follow-up over 5 years	Self-reported	Medical records	RR = 4.3 (95% CI 0.6–5.8)	■ Prospective design ensures temporality ■ Case ascertainment via medical records limits misclassification of outcome; any outcome misclassification would be non-differential given the study design	■ Strong potential for selection bias due to loss to follow-up ■ Strong potential for non-differential misclassification of exposure given self-reported BMI ■ Limited statistical power ■ Insufficient follow-up time (5 years) for new dementia cases to be diagnosed	Good

(Continued)

Table 10.1 (*Continued*)

Author (year) study design	Study population	BMI at age 50 (exposure)	Dementia (outcome)	Main result	Key strengths	Key limitations	Quality
Author C (2023) **Prospective cohort**	1,000,000 randomly selected participants enrolled at age 50 and followed until death, with 99% follow-up over 30 years	Measured by research nurse at enrollment	Extended clinical interviews and cognitive testing performed annually	BMI ≥ 30 kg/m² vs < 30 kg/m² RR = 1.5 (95% CI 1.2–1.8)	▪ Prospective design ensures temporality ▪ Case ascertainment uses gold standard methodology, making any misclassification very unlikely ▪ Large sample size with long follow-up provides excellent statistical power ▪ Exposure measurement uses gold-standard approach and prevents misclassification ▪ High follow-up rate makes selection bias very unlikely	▪ None noted	Excellent

You might even want to add a column to note how you rated each article's overall quality (see Chapter 9 for approaches to assessing article quality). It is also helpful to sort the studies in a logical way; typically, organizing by study design and/or chronologically is helpful. What you include in the table is ultimately up to you—the goal is to make it easy for you to see the key information and identify patterns (or, lack thereof). Often, these tables are included in literature reviews as a way of providing readers with an easily accessible summary of the articles.

In the table cells, keep your descriptions brief and limited to the very key details. In other words, don't repeat everything from your STAR templates. You'll still want to have those handy as you start writing so that you can access the full details. The point of the table is to provide you with a visual summary of each study and to help you identify similarities and differences quickly and easily.

Often, you will notice patterns when you look at the information in a table that you might not have noticed otherwise. For example, you might observe that all the case-control studies report significant positive associations, while the prospective cohort studies find no statistically significant associations. Or, perhaps you notice that the studies that measure the exposure using self-report don't observe any significant association with the outcome, while those that measure the exposure using a clinical assessment do. Or, you might even see that the studies are so different from one another, that they really are not comparable. All of these situations (among others) would be important to recognize as you work to synthesize findings across the studies and come to an overall conclusion.

How do I put all this different information together?

Remember that your goal is to consider all the articles on a given topic and put their findings into context with one another. This task requires you to compare and contrast the articles' strengths and limitations, paying close attention to how methodologic differences might explain any observed differences in reported associations.

You can follow the process shown in Figure 10.2 to help you synthesize across the various studies. Once you have carefully read and critically analyzed each article,

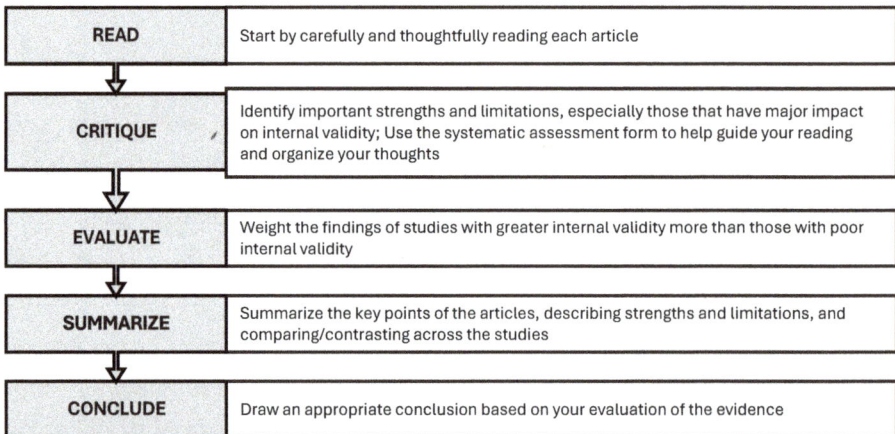

READ	Start by carefully and thoughtfully reading each article
CRITIQUE	Identify important strengths and limitations, especially those that have major impact on internal validity; Use the systematic assessment form to help guide your reading and organize your thoughts
EVALUATE	Weight the findings of studies with greater internal validity more than those with poor internal validity
SUMMARIZE	Summarize the key points of the articles, describing strengths and limitations, and comparing/contrasting across the studies
CONCLUDE	Draw an appropriate conclusion based on your evaluation of the evidence

Figure 10.2 Process for synthesizing results of epidemiologic articles that address a similar research question.

you want to weight the findings from studies with greater internal validity (i.e., the higher quality studies) more heavily than you weight those with poor internal validity (i.e., the lower quality studies). As you begin this exercise, it is important to remember that there is rarely a single correct conclusion; there are no easy answers, and even experts can disagree. Again, there are many different approaches to evaluating the quality of articles. The rating I give an article might differ from yours, for example, if you and I put a different emphasis on one study's strengths or the other study's limitations. Your goal is to come to your own conclusion and support that conclusion with a thoughtful critical analysis of the articles, both separately and together.

The following steps are likely to be helpful to you when comparing and contrasting across multiple studies:

1. For each study, identify the *most important* strengths and limitations that relate to the study population. Do you notice any similarities or differences in results that seem to track with similarities or differences, or strengths and limitations, of the study populations?
2. Compare and contrast the methods of *exposure measurement* across the studies: what are the strengths and limitations of the various approaches? How are the approaches similar or different? Are some approaches more valid than others? Do you notice any similarities or differences in results that seem to track with similarities or differences, or strengths and limitations, of the exposure measurement?
3. Compare and contrast the methods of *outcome measurement* across the studies: what are the strengths and limitations of the various approaches? How are the approaches similar or different? Are some approaches more valid than others? Do you notice any similarities or differences in results that seem to track with similarities or differences, or strengths and limitations, of the outcome measurement?
4. Which studies are of the highest quality? What makes them higher quality than the others? Do they find similar associations, or are they different? How might the strengths and/or limitations of the articles explain their similar (or different) findings?
5. Based on all of the above, what can you conclude about the research question being evaluated by all the studies?

Can you give me an example of how I could write all this up concisely?

Absolutely! Let's take a look at the hypothetical studies we summarized in Table 10.1, which have some pretty obvious differences among them.

We identified three (entirely made-up!) epidemiologic studies evaluating whether BMI at age 50 is associated with dementia later in life. Author A (2015) reported a small case-control study that recruited dementia cases (N = 100) from a local hospital and controls (N = 100) from among faculty and staff at a university in a neighboring state. Participants self-reported their BMI at age 50 and whether or not they had dementia. A strong positive association between BMI at age 50 and dementia was reported (OR 5.0, 95% CI 1.2–9.5). However, there are numerous limitations that diminish the study's internal validity. First, the study population has a strong potential for selection bias, especially given that the cases and controls were recruited from entirely separate source populations. Further, the age distributions of cases and controls are very likely to be very different, thus raising the possibility of confounding. Additionally, the retrospective design and self-report of exposure and outcome raise many issues. There is a major potential for recall bias, given that those with dementia may be particularly unable to accurately report their BMI at age 50 (exposure) or whether or not they have dementia (outcome). The statistical power is low, as evidenced by the small number of cases and controls as well as the wide confidence interval.

Author B (2019) also reported a strong positive association (RR 4.3, 95% CI 0.6–5.8). This study was a prospective cohort that followed 1,000 older adults recruited from the senior center; however, only 35% were followed up for dementia outcomes over 5 years. There is a major potential for selection bias to have occurred, especially if we believe that BMI may cause dementia and that those with dementia would be least likely to complete follow-up. This study also measured BMI at age 50 via self-report, which leaves a substantial opportunity for misclassification. Because of the prospective cohort design, however, the misclassification would most likely be non-differential and tend to bias results toward a null association. Medical records were used to measure dementia, which is a highly valid approach and minimizes the opportunity for non-differential and differential misclassification. Because a small (N = 1,000) cohort was originally enrolled and the follow-up rate was low, there were likely few dementia diagnoses recorded; statistical power was limited; as a result, again leading to a wide confidence interval.

The most recent study, Author C (2023), was a very large (N = 1,000,000) prospective cohort study that enrolled participants at age 50 and followed them until death, achieving a 99% follow-up rate over 30 years. There is almost no chance that selection bias would impact results, given that the participants were randomly selected and nearly all were followed up until death. Exposure was measured by a research nurse at the exact age needed for the exposure (BMI at age 50), which minimizes any opportunity for even non-differential misclassification. Further, the method of outcome ascertainment was outstanding: an extended clinical interview and cognitive testing were conducted with each participant annually to measure incident dementia. This is the gold-standard approach to diagnosing dementia, leaving little opportunity for outcome misclassification. The very large sample size generated a sufficient number of dementia cases and provided ample statistical power. This study reported that a BMI in the obese range at age 50, compared to a lower BMI, was associated with a 50% increased risk of dementia (RR 1.5, 95% CI 1.2–1.8).

Overall, the highest quality study was by Author C (2023); this study was rigorously designed and executed, with a study design and exposure and outcome assessment that significantly enhanced its internal validity. Selection bias likely substantially affects the estimated associations from the Author A (2015) and Author B (2019) studies, while this is not a concern in the Author C study. The approach to measuring exposure, especially, was far more valid in the Author C (2023) study as compared to the other studies, which relied on self-reported BMI and created major opportunities for non-differential and/or differential exposure misclassification. Outcome assessment and statistical power also were far stronger in the Author C study as compared to the other two. Although both the Author A and Author B studies reported strong, positive associations, neither was statistically significant and both studies have many serious threats to their internal validity. The most appropriate conclusion considering these three studies is that obesity at age 50 increases dementia risk by approximately 50%; this conclusion is supported by the rigorous and highly valid report of Author C (2023). Future research to confirm this finding is needed, however.

Activities

Find at least two additional articles that address a research question similar to the one explored in the article you read for the Activities in prior chapters (Chapters 3, 5–9).

1. Create a table that summarizes the key methodologic features, strengths, and limitations of each article, similar to Table 10.1.
2. Follow the process described in this chapter to compare and contrast across these articles, focusing on how similarities and differences in the key methodologic components (i.e., study design, study population, exposure assessment, and outcome assessment) impact internal validity and track with similarities and differences across the studies' results.
3. Based on the above, determine which studies are the highest quality, and form an overall conclusion about the research question under study.

CHAPTER 11

How do I perform a systematic literature review?

At this point, you have learned how to critically analyze individual epidemiologic articles and compare and contrast the results of studies on a similar topic. Because a single study is never definitive, evaluating all the existing literature on a given topic is important for arriving at an overall, evidence-based conclusion. This is of great importance whether you are seeking to decide what cancer screening to recommend to your patient or you are trying to identify the most effective intervention to promote physical activity in your community.

Enter the systematic literature review. As the name "systematic" suggests, this type of literature review uses pre-determined and objective methodology to identify, select, and evaluate epidemiologic articles that address a stated research question. Systematic literature reviews are highly important for synthesizing current knowledge in a field, identifying gaps to be targeted in future research, and supporting evidence-based decision-making for policy, patient care, and public health programs.

In this chapter, we will explore the standard approach for performing a systematic literature review. Drawing on the skills you have developed in critically analyzing individual articles and synthesizing the results of a group of articles, we will see how the systematic literature review utilizes an objective approach to ensure a truly scientific and objective assessment of the current state of knowledge on a given topic.

How is a systematic literature review different from narrative or scoping reviews?

You are likely already familiar with the term "literature review," and perhaps you have even read a number of these. Literature reviews are a specific type of scientific article that aims to explore and summarize the published (and sometimes even unpublished) body of knowledge on a topic. There are several ways to approach this.

One option is a **narrative review**, where the goal is to provide the reader with a broad understanding of what is known. For example, a recent narrative review of

DOI: 10.4324/9781003637899-12

the epidemiology of triple-negative breast cancer, a particularly aggressive subtype, summarizes what is known about a wide variety of risk factors and describes important disparities in its incidence.[1] If you are looking to quickly get up to speed in a field that is new to you, narrative reviews are generally quite helpful, as they provide a broad perspective of what is known. However, because the selection and inclusion of articles are entirely at the authors' discretion, narrative reviews are insufficient for supporting evidence-based decision-making. There is a possibility that some articles might be missed, and other articles might be intentionally left out because their findings do not support a pre-determined view. If you truly want to make evidence-based judgments, you need an objective approach to identifying and evaluating *all* the evidence.

The **scoping review** is increasingly popular, helped by the development of a formal methodology for this type of review. If we picture literature review approaches as a continuum, we can think of a scoping review as falling somewhere in between the narrative review and the systematic review. Scoping reviews aim to identify all the articles published on a given topic, helping the reader to understand the full scope of what is known. Many scoping reviews will include sources other than scientific articles (e.g., policy briefs). For example, a scoping review approach was used to explore how clinicians could avoid racial and ethnic discrimination when using clinical algorithms.[2] A scoping review, however, might not go into extensive detail on each published study and may or may not include critical analysis of the literature. Often, scoping reviews are used to identify gaps in the literature and/or to rigorously review the literature when it is too new to support a systematic review.[3]

Although scoping reviews are becoming more common, **systematic literature reviews** remain the preferred approach for epidemiologists. Systematic literature reviews truly are the foundation of evidence-based medicine and decision-making for policy, interventions, public health programs, and patient care. This type of literature review is used to synthesize current knowledge in a field, identify gaps to be addressed in future research, and identify common sources of bias and limitations. A systematic literature review uses a systematic (obviously), objective, and pre-determined approach to identify and evaluate *all* published studies on a given topic. By including all relevant research, systematic literature reviews are less prone to presenting a biased evaluation. For example, a recent systematic literature review and meta-analysis re-examined studies exploring associations between alcohol intake and mortality.[4] This careful analysis identified an issue with how prior studies had been analyzed that upended a prevailing view that low alcohol consumption was protective.

What are the steps for conducting a systematic literature review?

Typically, published systematic literature reviews involve the efforts of a team of researchers, with multiple investigators performing searches, abstracting information, and collaboratively writing up the results. But you can also perform a thorough systematic literature review on your own. You likely will need to have a narrower research question than if you were working as part of a larger research team, though, so that the number of articles remains manageable for a single individual.

There are many excellent, in-depth resources for learning about the methodology of a systematic literature review.[8–10] Here, I will give a high-level overview of the steps that

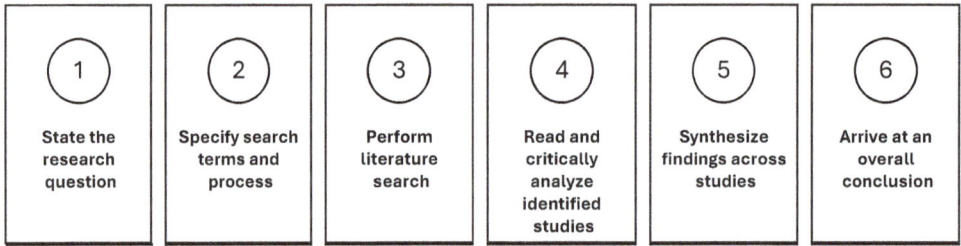

Figure 11.1 Steps for conducting a systematic literature review.

are involved. You can think of a systematic literature review as an epidemiologic study where the unit of observation is the scientific article, rather than an individual participant. But just like an observational study or randomized controlled trial, we need to think carefully about—and thoroughly document—the methods we use to conduct the study. Here, the methods refer to how the articles were identified, how the information from each one was abstracted and evaluated, and any tools that were used to evaluate bias and synthesize results.

Essentially, you can break the process of conducting a systematic literature review into a series of six steps (Figure 11.1). Let's consider each of these steps in turn.

Step 1: State the research question

The first step to conducting a systematic literature review is to clearly articulate the research question you are trying to answer. Don't be fooled into thinking that this step will be simple or quick. You will want to spend time making sure that your research question uses very precise language to clearly specify what you want to evaluate. For example, the research question "is physical activity related to heart disease?" is too broad. Will the review focus on risk of heart disease, or on survival from heart disease? And, what is meant by "heart disease"? Will the review focus on myocardial infarction, coronary heart disease, or some other disease or condition? A more specific and appropriately focused research question might be, "does physical activity affect risk of incident myocardial infarction?"

There are some frameworks available to help researchers articulate their questions for systematic literature reviews. For example, reviews of clinical topics (e.g., treatments, interventions) often phrase research questions by specifying the population, intervention, comparison, and outcome (PICO), while epidemiological studies might be better framed around population, exposure, outcome (PEO).[11] Following one of these frameworks can be helpful in specifying an appropriately focused research question to guide your search process.

Typically, generating the research question is an iterative process. Researchers generate a question based on what they already know about the topic, likely even performing a preliminary literature search (see Step 2), reviewing those results, and then refining the research question as needed. The goal is to channel our inner Goldilocks and find the research question that is just right; in other words, the one that is neither too broad nor too narrow.

Step 2: Specify search terms and process

The next step is to determine how you will find articles to answer your research question. What databases will you search? What search terms will you use? How will you know if an article should be included or not? Working with a librarian at your institution is often very helpful for developing your search methodology.

There are many databases that could be used for searching for relevant articles; some of these may require paid subscription, so check your institution's library for databases available to you. PubMed (https://pubmed.ncbi.nlm.nih.gov) is a free, publicly available database that includes millions of epidemiologic and biomedical articles. Even with the proliferation of other databases, PubMed remains a favorite among epidemiologists and medical professionals. Whatever database(s) you use, be sure to clearly document them, as this is a key part of the methods for your literature review.

Once you've identified databases, you'll need to come up with a list of search terms to use. Scanning the list of medical subject headings (MeSH)[12] that is compiled by the National Library of Medicine can be helpful, as databases like PubMed will tag articles using these terms. Often, researchers start a systematic literature review with a few articles in mind. Looking at the MeSH terms for those articles can be a good starting point for generating your list of search terms.

Beyond searching databases, there are other ways to identify relevant articles. For example, checking the citation lists of articles that you identify through database searching can be a useful approach for finding additional articles. Or, if you are looking for randomized controlled trials and are concerned about possible publication bias, you could look at clinicaltrials.gov to identify results from studies that may not have been published.

You will need to specify all inclusion and exclusion criteria to identify articles that are eligible for the systematic literature review. For example, you might only be interested in studies of humans, or in studies that examine mortality from the disease. For systematic literature reviews on topics that have a vast literature, researchers might include only studies using a certain study design (e.g., prospective cohort study) or that were published in the past 5 years.

As with formulating your research question, developing the search methodology is an iterative process. Typically, researchers will test their search terms and eligibility criteria and fine-tune their methods before moving on to the next step.

Step 3: Perform the literature search

Now it's (finally) time to perform the literature search. It is important to keep good documentation for every step of the search. How many articles were identified initially? How many were excluded, and for what reasons? How many articles were ultimately selected for inclusion in the review? It's helpful to think about, and perhaps even draft, a flow chart as you go. In the next section, we will learn about a recommended format for these figures; you can easily create your own flow chart following these guidelines by using a free web-based tool.[7]

You will also want to keep good records of every article you considered and why it was included or excluded. A simple spreadsheet can be immensely useful for this task, although other more sophisticated software applications to facilitate systematic literature reviews are available as well (e.g., Rayyan, a free online tool[13]).

When you enter your search terms into the database and apply any appropriate filters, you will likely generate a long list of potentially eligible articles. Next, you'll need to screen each article to see whether it fits your specified inclusion and exclusion criteria. A good first step is to screen each article's Title, excluding those that clearly do not fit the eligibility criteria. For example, if your research question specifies "death from myocardial infarction," then an article title that focuses only on risk of myocardial infarction would not be eligible. Or, if only randomized controlled trials are eligible, then an article title identifying the study design as case-control would be excluded.

Once you've narrowed down your initial list of articles, you then should read the Abstract of each remaining article. Here again, you are looking for clear evidence that the study is eligible or not eligible, documenting any articles you decide to exclude along with the reason(s). Finally, you will retrieve the full text of all remaining articles and examine their Methods section to verify their eligibility. This final set of articles becomes the dataset for your systematic literature review.

Step 4: Read and critically analyze identified articles

Once we have identified the final articles for inclusion in the systematic literature review, it's time to read and critically analyze each one. It is important to carefully abstract information about the study design, population, exposure, and outcome as well as the primary results. Keeping the details of multiple articles straight will be nearly impossible if you don't take good notes. Here, the STAR template (Appendix A) will be quite helpful. If you are unsure about how to read and critically analyze the individual articles, then take some time to review the earlier chapters of this book.

Step 5: Synthesize findings across articles

Now, it is time to put it all together. This is where the concepts covered in Chapter 10 come into play (if you haven't read Chapter 10 yet, now would be a good time to do so). It is important to put the results into context with one another, carefully considering how the results are similar or different, the various strengths and limitations of each study, and weighing the results from the studies deemed to have highest internal and external validity more than those that are substantially impacted by bias, confounding and error. Create a table following the format of Table 10.1 to summarize the key information across the articles. This table will be extremely useful as you move on to the final step in conducting a systematic literature review.

Step 6: Arrive at an overall conclusion

Now that you have completed a thorough critical analysis of each article and compared across the articles, it is time to arrive at your overall conclusion. Again, refer back to the discussion within Chapter 10 for arriving at an overall conclusion based on the critical analysis of multiple articles on a given topic. If you performed a meta-analysis as part of the systematic literature review, then the summary measure of association will be helpful here. Either way, your overall conclusion should incorporate answers to the following questions: Based on everything you've read, what is the most appropriate answer to the specified research question? What gaps and/or common biases did you note? What needs to be done next?

What is PRISMA?

PRISMA stands for Preferred Reporting Items of Systematic Reviews and Meta-Analyses.[5] Like the CONSORT and STROBE statements that established guidelines for reporting randomized controlled trials and observational studies, respectively, PRISMA is a widely accepted standard for reporting systematic literature reviews. The PRISMA statement was originally published in 2009 and updated in 2020. PRISMA specifies what should be reported in a written systematic literature review as well as how that information should be reported. By establishing reporting guidelines for systematic literature reviews, the PRISMA statement enhances the quality of such articles (assuming they follow the guidelines, of course). Most high-quality peer-reviewed journals now require authors to follow the PRISMA guidelines for all published systematic literature reviews.

The essence of the PRISMA statement is a checklist of twenty-seven items to be reported along with a flow chart to document the entire process of searching and selecting articles for inclusion. The PRISMA website (www.prisma-statement.org) includes the complete PRISMA statement as well as editable versions of the PRISMA checklist and flowchart.

The checklist specifies information that should be reported in each section of the systematic literature review, including the Title (explicitly state the article is a systematic review), the Introduction (e.g., articulate a clear objective), the Methods (e.g., identify eligibility criteria for selecting articles), the Results (e.g., describe potential for bias in each study), and Discussion (e.g., synthesize and evaluate evidence), as well as other information that should be reported (e.g., stating conflicts of interest).

Perhaps the most recognizable feature of PRISMA is the flow chart (Figure 11.2) that summarizes the entire search process from start to finish. This graphical display clearly identifies the databases and search terms used, the number of articles reviewed, all reasons for exclusion of articles, the number of articles excluded, and the final number of eligible and included articles.

What is the difference between pooling and meta-analysis?

You may have come across review articles that describe pooling data or performing a meta-analysis. It is important to recognize that these are two distinct approaches. While they are both ways of combining information across multiple studies on a given topic, the methodology they use to accomplish this is quite different.

In a **pooled analysis**, the investigators obtain the individual-level data from each of the studies and combine them into a single dataset. This has the effect of substantially increasing the sample size and, thus, statistical power. The estimated measure of association from a pooled analysis, therefore, will be more precise (i.e., have a narrower confidence interval) than that from the individual studies. Pooled analyses are particularly helpful for research questions that involve truly rare outcomes, as individual studies may each have insufficient statistical power on their own. For example, a recent pooled analysis evaluated whether talc causes ovarian cancer; by combining data from eight different case-control studies, researchers were able to assemble a dataset including 8,525 cases and 9,589 controls. The pooled analysis facilitated a highly powered analysis, resulting in the identification of a statistically significant, small increased risk of ovarian cancer associated with genital powder use (OR 1.23, 95% CI 1.15–1.33).[14]

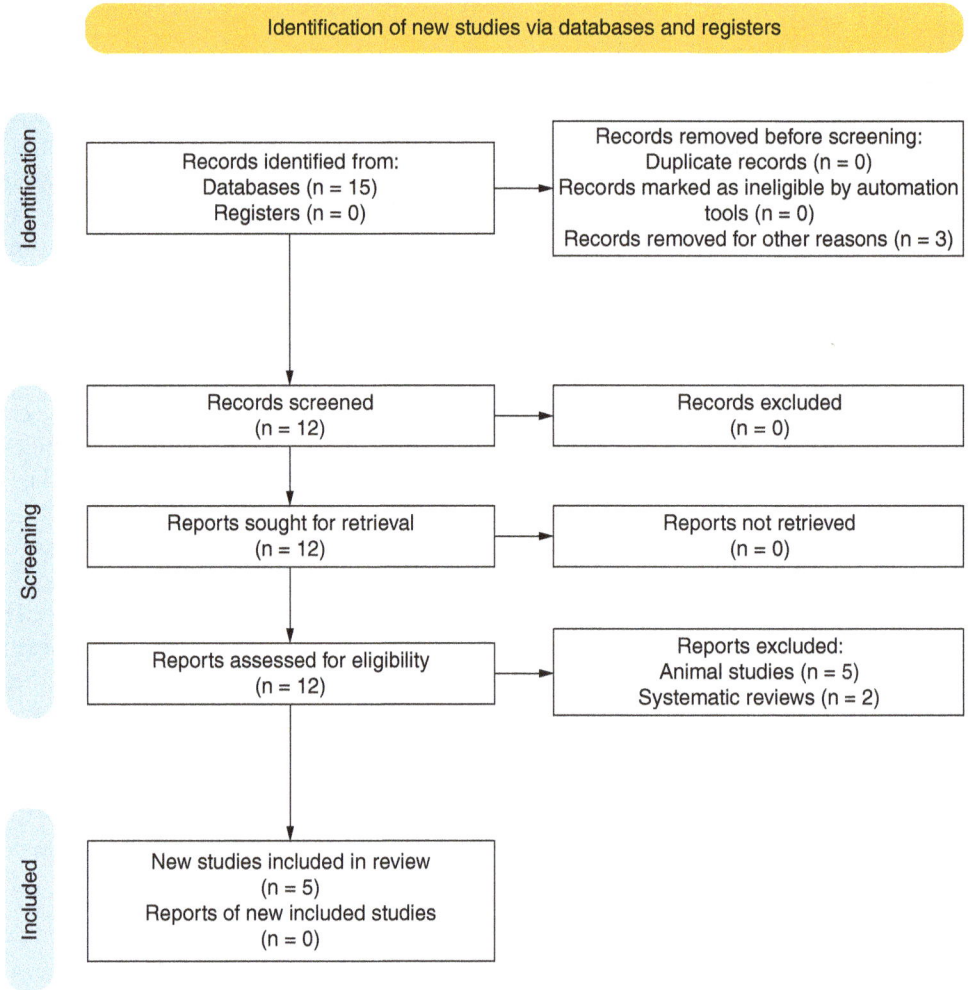

Figure 11.2 Example of a PRISMA flow chart showing the search and screening process used in a previously published systematic literature review,[6] created using an online tool.[7] Licensed under CC BY 4.0. Modified by Katherine W. Reeves. (https://www.eshackathon.org/software/PRISMA2020.html).

Pooled analyses can be quite challenging to conduct. First, researchers must obtain access to the individual studies' data, which often involves forming a consortium and securing funding to support the research. The biggest challenge, though, often comes with the need to harmonize the data across studies. As we have seen, there are many different ways of measuring a single exposure, outcome, or other key variable. In order to pool data across the studies, the investigators must harmonize these approaches, making them as similar as possible. For example, the pooled analysis of genital powder use and ovarian cancer noted that each study had its own definition of exposure, with some defining use as ever/never and others defining use for at least a year as regular use.[14]

Study	OR/RR	OR/RR	95%-CI	Weight
Author A		5.00	[0.65; 9.35]	0.5%
Author B		4.30	[1.70; 6.90]	1.3%
Author C		1.50	[1.20; 1.80]	98.2%
Common effect model		1.55	[1.26; 1.85]	100.0%

-5   0   5
Effect Size

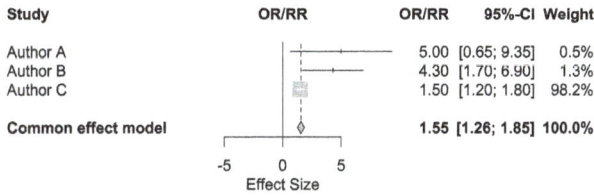

Figure 11.3 Example Forest plot showing a meta-analysis for the hypothetical studies summarized in Table 10.1.

A **meta-analysis** similarly has the goal of combining information across multiple studies to create a single overall measure of the exposure-outcome association. A meta-analysis essentially calculates a weighted average of measures of association obtained from individual studies. The unit of observation in a meta-analysis becomes the study itself, whereas the unit of observation in a pooled analysis remains individual participants. Because there is no need to request individual-level data from study investigators, a meta-analysis may be more feasible to perform than a pooled analysis.

Many systematic literature reviews will incorporate a meta-analysis, but not all do. Often, meta-analyses will summarize their findings in a useful figure referred to as a **Forest plot**. A Forest plot (Figure 11.3.) graphically displays the measures of association and confidence intervals estimated from each individual study along with the overall, summary estimate. When possible, meta-analyses will often calculate summary estimates including only studies with a certain design (e.g., prospective cohort studies) or that were judged to have the highest quality.

A limitation of meta-analyses, however, is that methodology across studies may be so different that we are not really making apples-to-apples comparisons, and thus, combining results across very different studies may not be appropriate. Because data are not harmonized, it can be challenging to interpret the results of a meta-analysis when the underlying studies defined exposure or outcome very differently. Also, if present, publication bias (see Chapter 1) can impact the findings of meta-analyses. Research teams conducting meta-analyses often invest a great deal of effort in finding unpublished work to include and ensure the summary estimate generated by the meta-analysis represents an unbiased estimate of the association being evaluated.

Where can I find rigorous systematic literature reviews on medical topics?

You might have realized by now that conducting a systematic literature review requires substantial effort, often involving a team of investigators working together over months or even years. The good news is that you don't have to conduct your own systematic literature review every time you want an evidence-based answer to an important question. Because conducting a rigorous systematic literature review, with or without a meta-analysis, takes an extraordinary amount of time, it would be highly impractical to perform one yourself before every policy recommendation or treatment decision. So, how can you find a published systematic literature review that you can trust?

One option is to use PubMed to search for a systematic literature review on your topic. This is typically the preferred approach for epidemiologists and other researchers. PubMed includes a filter to restrict the results list to include only systematic literature reviews. While PubMed is great for identifying a systematic literature review, it leaves the evaluation of the review quality entirely up to you. We can evaluate the quality of a systematic literature review by (1) checking if the article follows the PRISMA reporting guidelines, (2) using our critical analysis skills to think through the strengths and limitations of the included articles, and (3) deciding if the authors' conclusions align with our own evaluation. This can be time-consuming, though, and there also may not be a systematic literature review on every topic of interest.

Many medical and healthcare practitioners instead prefer to use databases that were created for the explicit purpose of evaluating and summarizing scientific literature to support evidence-based decision-making. There are many of these out there, but I'll mention two that seem to be both popular and of high quality (which hopefully is what has made them so popular!).

The Cochrane Library (https://www.cochranelibrary.com/) is a non-profit organization based in the United Kingdom that produces a collection of databases to evaluate and synthesize scientific evidence for medical and healthcare professionals. This group conducts its own systematic literature reviews. These are available in the *Cochrane Database of Systematic Reviews,* along with written protocols for how the reviews are conducted.

Another option is UpToDate® (https://www.wolterskluwer.com/en/solutions/uptodate), which includes rigorous evaluation of scientific literature to support clinical care and drug decisions. The reviews included in UpToDate® are most accurately described as scoping reviews, but they are generally viewed as rigorous and of high quality. Medical professionals especially appreciate the integration with many electronic health record systems, such that they can easily find answers to their clinical questions when needed.

Whatever the source of the systematic literature review, however, you should still take the time to thoroughly read and critically evaluate the article. As you have seen with other types of epidemiologic studies and articles, you may not always agree with the authors' conclusions. And, even excellent journals or reputable databases sometimes publish articles that are later corrected or discredited. As students, researchers, and health professionals, you should always value your own evaluation of the evidence.

Activities

Find a recent systematic literature review that was published on a topic of interest to you. You may wish to find one related to the topic of the article you've used to complete the Activities in the previous chapters.

1. Use the PRISMA checklist to assess how well the review adheres to the PRISMA guidelines.
2. Perform a literature search using the methods described in the article. Were you able to reproduce the search results described in the article? How might you improve the search strategy that was used?

3. Read and critically analyze any relevant epidemiologic articles that were not included in the original systematic literature review, especially those that were published after the review. Compare and contrast these studies to those that were included. Do they confirm the conclusions of the systematic literature review, or do they provide a new perspective?

References

1. Howard F, Olopade O. Epidemiology of triple-negative breast cancer: A review. *Cancer J.* 2021;27(1): 8–16. doi:10.1097/PPO.0000000000000500
2. Cary MP, Zink A, Wei S, et al. Mitigating racial and ethnic bias and advancing health equity in clinical algorithms: A scoping review. *Health Aff.* 2023;42(10):1359–1368. doi:10.1377/hlthaff.2023.00553
3. Munn Z, Peters MDJ, Stern C, Tufanaru C, McArthur A, Aromataris E. Systematic review or scoping review? Guidance for authors when choosing between a systematic or scoping review approach. *BMC Med Res Methodol.* 2018;18(1):143. doi:10.1186/s12874-018-0611-x
4. Zhao J, Stockwell T, Naimi T, Churchill S, Clay J, Sherk A. Association between daily alcohol intake and risk of all-cause mortality: A systematic review and meta-analyses. *JAMA Netw Open.* 2023;6(3):e236185. doi:10.1001/jamanetworkopen.2023.6185
5. Page MJ, McKenzie JE, Bossuyt PM, et al. The PRISMA 2020 statement: An updated guideline for reporting systematic reviews. *BMJ.* 2021;372:n71. doi:10.1136/bmj.n71
6. Heilmann NZ, Reeves KW, Hankinson SE. Phthalates and bone mineral density: A systematic review. *Environ Health Glob Access Sci Source.* 2022;21(1):108. doi:10.1186/s12940-022-00920-5
7. Haddaway NR, Page MJ, Pritchard CC, McGuinness LA. *PRISMA2020*: An R package and Shiny app for producing PRISMA 2020-compliant flow diagrams, with interactivity for optimised digital transparency and open synthesis. *Campbell Syst Rev.* 2022;18(2):e1230. doi:10.1002/cl2.1230
8. Cochrane Handbook for Systematic Reviews of Interventions. Accessed September 20, 2024. https://training.cochrane.org/handbook
9. Dekkers OM, Vandenbroucke JP, Cevallos M, Renehan AG, Altman DG, Egger M. COSMOS-E: Guidance on conducting systematic reviews and meta-analyses of observational studies of etiology. *PLoS Med.* 2019;16(2):e1002742. doi:10.1371/journal.pmed.1002742
10. IOM (Institute of Medicine). 2011. Finding What Works in Health Care: Standards for Systematic Reviews. Washington, DC: The National Academies Press. https://doi.org/10.17226/13059.
11. Cantrell S. LibGuides: Systematic Reviews: 2. Develop a Research Question. Accessed September 20, 2024. https://guides.mclibrary.duke.edu/sysreview/question
12. Medical Subject Headings - Home Page. Accessed September 20, 2024. https://www.nlm.nih.gov/mesh/meshhome.html
13. Rayyan – Intelligent Systematic Review - Rayyan. November 8, 2021. Accessed September 20, 2024. https://www.rayyan.ai/
14. Terry KL, Karageorgi S, Shvetsov YB, et al. Genital powder use and risk of ovarian cancer: A pooled analysis of 8,525 cases and 9,859 controls. *Cancer Prev Res.* 2013;6(8):811–821. doi:10.1158/1940–6207.CAPR-13–0037

Why can't I just use artificial intelligence (AI) to critically analyze epidemiologic articles?

This is a fair question. If you have read this far into the book, you are probably already convinced that you need to develop critical analysis skills for yourself. But, the rapid improvements in generative artificial intelligence (AI) are clearly changing how we all work and the skills we will need to be successful in our careers. You can now obtain a summary of any article—or even of all published articles on a given topic—in a matter of seconds. It's reasonable to think that the days of manually searching through PubMed for articles on your research question are over (or, at least, permanently changed). It's a totally new world.

It would be foolhardy of me to tell you to never use AI tools. AI is not going away. The reality is that (1) you probably already are using them, (2) your current or future workplaces will expect you to use them, and (3) they can actually be very helpful. But it would also be wrong for me not to warn you about the potential pitfalls of AI. AI will get you the answer quickly, but the answer you get won't always be right. If you don't have a firm grounding in all of the concepts we've discussed in this book to this point, you will lack the ability to distinguish between fact and "hallucination."

So, to answer the question posed by the chapter title, you actually *could* use AI tools to critically analyze epidemiologic articles. The issue is that they likely won't do a very good job. Of course, AI technology is evolving so rapidly that we can anticipate it will continue to improve its capabilities in the near future. Even so, you will always need to understand the strengths and limitations of epidemiologic articles for yourself. You will need strong critical analysis skills to make sound judgments about what therapy to recommend for your patients or to ask innovative questions in your research. While you shouldn't expect AI to fully replace your own thinking, you also shouldn't expect that you won't use it at all. You need to work in partnership with AI.

DOI: 10.4324/9781003637899-13

What is AI?

First, I should let you know that I am by no means an expert in this area. I'm learning all this in real time, just like you are. Rather than do a subpar job of defining AI myself, I decided to go straight to the source. That's right—I asked ChatGPT to define AI for me[1]:

> **Artificial Intelligence (AI)** is a field of computer science focused on creating machines that can perform tasks typically requiring human intelligence. These tasks include recognizing patterns, making decisions, learning from experience, understanding natural language, and even solving complex problems. Think of AI as teaching computers to think and act in ways that mimic human abilities, but often with much greater speed and accuracy.

When ChatGPT arrived on the scene in late 2022, it immediately changed the way all different types of tasks could be done. Suddenly, entire papers could be "written" in a matter of seconds. It's probably safe for me to assume that you have already used AI, either in your personal or professional life. Perhaps you've even used it to support your academic work.

Like many things in life, the quality of what you will get out of an AI tool generally matches the quality of what you put into it. The **prompt** refers to the set of instructions you give to the AI tool. The better your prompt is, the better response the AI tool will produce. Writing an effective AI prompt is an important skill to develop, and future workers (and maybe even students!) will be expected to know how to do this well. You will get the best results from an AI application when you specify (1) the task you want it to complete, (2) the format its response should take, (3) the voice in which the response should be written, and (4) the context in which the prompt is being asked.[2]

For example, I generated the above definition of AI using the following prompt: *Write a concise definition of AI for a textbook written in a conversational tone for an educated audience.* Notice how I specified the task (write a definition), the format (concise), the voice (conversational), and the context (a textbook for an educated audience). If you aren't happy with the result the AI tool gives you initially, try modifying your prompt. Working with the AI tool in an iterative process will give you a better result.

What are the potential advantages of using AI?

It is quite clear that AI can speed up your work significantly. It is completely realistic to think that the days of scrolling through PubMed hits and scanning hundreds of titles to find relevant literature might be over. AI has the potential to make your literature search process both faster and more thorough. In fact, we will explore an AI tool, Research Rabbit, that already does this fairly well, later in this chapter.

AI is good at writing summaries of articles, although the quality of these summaries varies markedly across AI tools. You could even ask the AI tool to change the voice in which a summary is written. For example, you might want a summary written without using technical jargon if you are new to a field. Reading AI-generated summaries could be a good way to learn background information on a new topic. When writing your critical analysis, you might find that AI can help by writing the article summary that begins the critical analysis paper, giving you more time to focus on the critical analysis piece itself. While you will still need to edit (and fact-check) the summary that the AI tool writes, it could be useful to help you get started.

What are the potential limitations of using AI?

Quick identification and summarizing of relevant articles seem like pretty great strengths. You might be wondering, "what's the catch?" Well, there are many catches. AI is good at summarizing, but its critical thinking skills are lackluster at best. This is one area where the human brain is (at least as of this writing) much better than the computer brain. It would definitely be faster to write your critical analysis using AI, but it won't be nearly as in-depth (or accurate) as you can write on your own. In their book exploring how AI is changing higher education, Bowen and Watson equate generative AI models to a C-level student.[2] Assuming you want to do far better than mediocre work, you will need to enhance any AI-generated output with your own human-generated critical analysis.

Generative AI tools produce text by predicting what words are most likely to come next, based on their database. As a result, they can repeat biases that are already in the literature. In other words, if the prevailing wisdom is that X causes Y, that is what AI is most likely to tell you. The AI will typically agree with whatever the authors of the article state as their conclusion, failing to carefully weigh the strengths and limitations and their impact on internal and external validity. In other words, the AI tool won't do any of the things you've spent the last eleven chapters learning how to do.

When synthesizing across multiple articles, AI also will treat each article as equally valid, which could mean that a study with very poor internal validity would contribute to the overall conclusion just as much as a study with very high internal validity. As discussed in Chapter 10, studies with higher internal validity need to be weighed more heavily than those with poorer internal validity as you evaluate the literature.

Importantly, AI often makes mistakes. In the AI world, these mistakes are called **hallucinations** and could include everything from inaccurately stating a fact to completely making up citations. If you ask AI to search the literature for you, it is possible that it might miss important studies or that it will include studies that didn't meet your criteria. If you want to use AI, you need to be able to recognize these hallucinations when they happen. But how can you recognize hallucinations if you can't critically analyze the article yourself? Fortunately, you have mastered these skills as you have worked your way through this book.

Could I use AI to write my critical analysis? A cautionary tale

Just because AI can generate a written critical analysis of an article in less than a minute doesn't mean that it will be any good. Below is a critical analysis of the Mirick et al.[3] article that I asked ChatGPT[4] to write for me (literally typing: *write a critical analysis of Mirick 2002 article on antiperspirants and breast cancer*):

> The 2002 JNCI article by Mirick et al titled "Antiperspirant Use and the Risk of Breast Cancer" sought to investigate the potential link between the use of

antiperspirants and breast cancer. While the study was well-intentioned, it had several limitations that raise questions about the validity of its findings.

One of the key issues with the study is its design. The study was a case-control study, which means that the researchers recruited women who had already been diagnosed with breast cancer and asked them to recall their use of antiperspirants in the past. This retrospective design can be subject to recall bias, as it relies on the accuracy of participants' memories. Participants may not accurately recall their use of antiperspirants, especially if they were diagnosed with breast cancer after many years of using the product.

Another issue with the study is that the researchers did not control for potential confounding factors that could influence the risk of breast cancer. For example, the study did not consider family history of breast cancer, age at menarche, age at first birth, or use of hormone replacement therapy. These factors are known to be associated with breast cancer risk, and failing to account for them could have introduced bias into the study's findings.

Additionally, the study had a relatively small sample size of just 437 women with breast cancer and 518 women without breast cancer. The small sample size limits the statistical power of the study, making it difficult to draw definitive conclusions.

The study's findings were also contradicted by other research on the topic. For example, a large cohort study published in the same year found no association between antiperspirant use and breast cancer risk. Furthermore, the National Cancer Institute has stated that there is no conclusive evidence linking antiperspirants to breast cancer.

In conclusion, while the 2002 JNCI article by Mirick et al provided an interesting hypothesis about the potential link between antiperspirant use and breast cancer, its limitations and inconsistencies with other research suggest that its findings should be interpreted with caution. More research is needed to better understand the potential risks associated with antiperspirant use and breast cancer.

While this might look like a decent critical analysis at first, upon closer inspection, there are some major issues, including:

- Lacks a brief, non-evaluative description of the study.
- Fails to identify and evaluate any strengths of the study.
- Notes limitations (e.g., "participants may not accurately recall their use of antiperspirants"), but does not explain how or why this would impact internal validity.
- Incorrectly states that the statistical analyses did not adjust for potential confounders.
- Reports incorrect sample sizes, describes the sample size as "relatively small," and raises concerns about statistical power. However, this concern is not supported with any calculations (I ran the calculations myself, and the authors had 80% power to detect the observed odds ratio).
- Fails to state the results of the study. In fact, it reads as if the study's results contradict the statement from the National Cancer Institute (NCI), while the findings of no association are actually in agreement (and NCI cites the Mirick study in their statement[5]).

■   Makes an overly general conclusion—it has a lot of words, but it doesn't say anything meaningful.

Although generative AI technology is rapidly improving, it remains an insufficient substitute for your own critical analysis and evaluation of epidemiologic articles.

How good are currently available AI tools for searching and summarizing scientific articles?

Numerous AI tools have been developed to support scientists in identifying and "reading" scientific articles. These tools will continue to improve, and I imagine that newer, better AI tools for this purpose will exist by the time this book is published. Keeping this in mind, it is still helpful to examine a few currently available tools: Consensus, Elicit, and Research Rabbit. I tested each one out using a similar prompt to see if they could help answer the question of whether antiperspirants cause breast cancer based on scientific evidence. Note that while these sites required me to register with them, the results were generated from the free versions of the tools.

Consensus (https://consensus.app)

In response to the research question "do antiperspirants cause breast cancer," Consensus provided a list of relevant articles and the following summary, based on ten papers, in response to my research question: "Some studies suggest antiperspirants do not increase the risk of breast cancer, while other studies suggest a potential link due to hormone exposure." Consensus also reported that of twelve papers analyzed, 0% said Yes, 25% said Possibly, and 75% said No.[6]

You likely noticed that the results of the synthesis summary and percentages of Yes/No/Possibly don't seem to agree. First, they are derived from a different number of articles (ten and twelve, respectively). Second, the summary indicates that the studies have truly mixed results, while the 75% rated as "No" indicates strong agreement that antiperspirants do not cause breast cancer.

Neither of these approaches to summarizing the identified literature weighed the study's findings by any measure of quality. The list of articles identified, however, did have article tags indicating if the article had been frequently cited or if it was published in a high-quality journal. The latter tag is a bit puzzling, though, as it was given to an article published in the *Journal of Cosmetic Dermatology*, which has an impact factor of 2.3, but not to an article published in the *Journal of the National Cancer Institute*, which has an impact factor of 9.9.[7]

Also, the list of articles returned included some articles that were not appropriate for answering the question of whether antiperspirants "cause" breast cancer. For example, the results list included a randomized controlled trial of antiperspirant use among breast cancer patients during their treatment. The list also included non-systematic literature reviews (including one written by McGrath, the author of the poor quality study we examined at the beginning of this book,[8] published in a journal titled *Medical Hypotheses*).

Consensus does give the option to filter results, and you could use that tool to restrict to only observational studies. Doing so, however, returned only three articles and did not materially change the summary: "Some studies suggest antiperspirant use does not increase the risk of breast cancer, while other studies suggest frequent use and under-arm shaving may be associated with an earlier age at diagnosis."[6]

Elicit (https://elicit.com)

Using the same research question, "do antiperspirants cause breast cancer," Elicit provided a table of relevant articles and a scientific-sounding summary[9]:

> The association between antiperspirant use and breast cancer risk has been investigated in several studies, with no evidence supporting a causal relationship. A population-based case-control study found no increased risk of breast cancer associated with antiperspirant or deodorant use (Mirick et al., 2002). Similarly, a study in Iraq reported no association between antiperspirant use and breast cancer risk (Fakri et al., 2006). A systematic review of observational studies concluded that there was insufficient evidence to conduct a quantitative analysis, emphasizing the need for further prospective studies (Allam, 2016). An expert group analyzed existing literature and found no scientific evidence supporting the hypothesis of a link between deodorants/antiperspirants and breast cancer, aligning with the conclusions of French, European, and American health authorities (Namer et al., 2008). Overall, current research does not support the claim that antiperspirant use increases breast cancer risk.

The free version of Elicit only generates summaries of up to four articles at once (although the paid versions allow you to summarize more).

Elicit provided the article list in the form of a summary table, similar to the one that I introduced in Chapter 10. The table initially included ten articles, though with the option to add more results by clicking a button at the bottom of the page (although the more I clicked that button, the less related the articles it returned became). Elicit's table included a citation to each article as well as a one-sentence summary of the Abstract; there was an option to add additional columns if you wanted (with the paid versions providing more columns). The option to add a column of limitations was a nice feature. However, there was a big caveat with the limitations Elicit identified: it was clear to me that Elicit was only basing the limitations on the article's Abstract. If you were to rely on Elicit to identify the limitations of an article for you, you would miss most of them.

Elicit did not evaluate article or journal quality, although it did show how many times an article had been cited. There was an option to filter results based on a quality metric, derived from a ranking system related to the number of citations a journal receives.

Additional filters were available to help narrow down the results. Before applying any filters, the article list generated for me included several articles that did not report results of primary research. For example, the results list included many literature reviews. There was a study-type filter that could be helpful in refining the results list, but it was not easy to restrict the articles to include only those that studied humans. More problematic, though, was that one of the articles returned by Elicit was not a primary research article but rather was a commentary written about a case-control study (even more surprising, the case-control study itself was not included in the results list). If you wanted to identify only observational epidemiologic studies, your best bet would be to review the complete article list yourself.

Research Rabbit (https://www.researchrabbit.ai/)

Research Rabbit is a very different AI tool than either Consensus or Elicit. It is designed to help researchers identify articles of interest, and it can be set up to search PubMed from within the Research Rabbit application. At the time I tested it out, this tool didn't generate article summaries. But, Research Rabbit did do a good job of finding relevant articles using PubMed. Instead of typing in my research question, I started by adding the Mirick et al. article to my collection in Research Rabbit.[10] From there, the tool generated a web that showed all the articles that had cited the Mirick et al.[3] article, as well as their connections (via citations) to one another; presumably, the ones closer to Mirick et al. might be the articles I'd be most interested in.

There were options to filter results, although the filtering appeared to be based on words appearing in the Title or Abstract. For example, asking Research Rabbit to restrict to human studies still returned some laboratory studies that happened to have the word "human" in the Title. This AI tool could make literature searching far more efficient and save you a lot of time, although you still would need to review the results to ensure that they meet whatever criteria you have specified.

How can I partner with AI when writing a critical analysis of article(s)?

The increased availability of software powered by AI is revolutionizing all facets of our daily and professional lives. AI is not going away, and, as I've said many times by now, it is only going to improve. The currently available tools I explored all have some things they do well, but also some areas of significant concern. As AI technology improves, though, so too will these types of tools.

While I am not categorically opposed to using AI, I strongly caution you against having it do all your work for you. AI might be helpful in improving your writing (especially if you are writing in a language other than your native language) or getting you unstuck from a severe case of writer's block. But, most academics would view handing in work that you did not write yourself as academic dishonesty. Many universities are updating their policies to include using AI in this way as a form of cheating.

Students might wonder if AI could be helpful in writing a critical analysis of an article. Hopefully, the cautionary tale I shared earlier has convinced you not to rely on AI for this purpose (unless, of course, you are ok with accepting a C grade). Future AI tools will likely be better at identifying relevant articles and summarizing their results. It seems unlikely, though, that AI will ever be able to replace the human ability to critically analyze these articles and put them into context with one another. And it certainly won't be able to render a conclusion that is influenced by your own unique perspective and set of values.

If you want to be successful as an epidemiologist or health professional (and if you've read this far into the book, I assume that you do), then you still will need to develop your critical analysis skills. AI is no substitute for your own thinking. Until AI can accurately identify strengths and limitations of articles (based on more than just the article's Abstract) and weigh the internal validity of the findings (by evaluating more than just the journal's reputation as a marker of quality), you will need to do this yourself. This is very good news—I certainly don't want a computer program to tell me what to think! I would, however, like one that can help me do my work more efficiently.

Our best approach to partnering with AI is to use it for what it does well. In my opinion, this includes literature searching (Research Rabbit has the potential to be very helpful for this) as well as writing initial drafts of article summaries (Elicit could be helpful here). Using AI in these ways will certainly save you a lot of time, allowing you to focus your effort on carefully reading and critically evaluating the article itself.

Activities

1. Use the AI tools described in this chapter to explore a research question of interest to you, perhaps the one you have explored in the previous chapters' activities. Evaluate the results they provide. How accurate are the summaries? Are relevant articles identified (and, are important articles excluded)? How well do these tools identify strengths and limitations and provide a critical analysis?
2. Read the policies of your favorite journal about the use of AI. Is AI addressed within their instructions to authors? Are there uses of AI that are specifically allowed, or specifically disallowed?
3. Interview your colleagues, instructors, and/or peers about their views on the use of AI within your profession. Are there uses that are acceptable (or, ones that are clearly unacceptable)? What patterns do you notice, if any, with how AI is viewed by people in different roles?

References

1. Open AI. Response generated by ChatGPT. *ChatGPT*, 2024. Accessed Aug 22 2024.
2. Bowen JA, Watson CE. *Teaching with AI: A Practical Guide to a New Era of Human Learning.* Johns Hopkins University Press; 2024.
3. Mirick DK, Davis S, Thomas DB. Antiperspirant use and the risk of breast cancer. *J Natl Cancer Inst.* 2002;94(20):1578–1580. doi:10.1093/jnci/94.20.1578
4. Open AI. Response generated by ChatGPT. *ChatGPT,* 2023. Accessed Apr 3 2023.
5. Antiperspirants/Deodorants and Breast Cancer - NCI. June 30, 2023. Accessed June 24, 2024. https://www.cancer.gov/about-cancer/causes-prevention/risk/myths/antiperspirants-fact-sheet
6. Consensus. Response generated by consensus. *Consensus*, 2024. Accessed Sept 3 2024.
7. Journal Citation Reports - Home. Accessed October 27, 2023. https://clarivate.com/products/scientific-and-academic-research/research-analytics-evaluation-and-management-solutions/journal-citation-reports/
8. McGrath KG. An earlier age of breast cancer diagnosis related to more frequent use of antiperspirants/deodorants and underarm shaving. *Eur J Cancer Prev.* 2003;12(6):479–485. doi:10.1097/00008469–200312000-00006
9. Elicit. Response generated by elicit. *Consensus*, 2024. Accessed Sept 3 2024.
10. Research Rabbit. Response generated by Research Rabbit. *Research Rabbit*, 2024. Accessed Sept 7 2024.

System for Taking notes on ARticles (STAR) Template

Full citation of journal article

1. Study purpose and design

Describe (i.e., report just the facts described in the article)	Critique (i.e., think through strengths/ limitations of the methods and results; address the key questions listed, and add additional comments as needed)
What is the objective/purpose of the study?	Is sufficient justification for the stated objective/ purpose provided? Is there a plausible biologic or theoretical mechanism provided?
What study design was used?	Is this an appropriate design for addressing the stated objective/purpose? Why or why not?
	Note any additional comments:

2. Study population

Describe (i.e., report just the facts described in the article)	Critique (i.e., think through strengths/ limitations of the methods and results; address the key questions listed, and add additional comments as needed)
What is the source population? Be specific—include geographic region, calendar time, age, race, ethnicity, sex, etc.	Is this an appropriate population in which to address the stated objective/purpose? Why or why not?
What eligibility criteria were specified?	Are these criteria appropriate? Why or why not?

(Continued)

(Continued)

2. Study population

How were participants selected and/or recruited?	Could the study results have been affected by selection bias? Did subject selection differ between comparison groups (i.e., differential loss-to-follow-up in exposed compared to unexposed in a cohort study; differential selection of cases compared to non-cases in a case-control study)?
	Were response/participation rates sufficient? Were they similar between comparison groups?
	To what larger population may the results of this study be generalized (e.g., the source population, additional groups)? If you include groups beyond the source population, justify why. If you think results couldn't be applied to certain groups, justify why.
	What other strengths and/or limitations do you note?

3. Exposure assessment

Describe (i.e., report just the facts described in the article)	Critique (i.e., think through strengths/limitations of the methods and results; address the key questions listed, and add additional comments as needed)
What was the primary exposure of interest?	Is this exposure appropriate for addressing the stated objective?
How was the primary exposure measured? Be specific—include details of measurement tools, assays, etc. used.	Was the measurement of exposure reliable? Was the measurement of exposure valid? What strengths and/or limitations do you note?
	Could the study results have been affected by **differential** misclassification of exposure? Why or why not? If so, describe direction, magnitude, and likelihood.
	Could the study results have been affected by **nondifferential** misclassification of the exposure? Why or why not? If so, describe direction, magnitude, and likelihood.
	Note any additional comments:

4. *Outcome assessment*

Describe (i.e., report just the facts described in the article)	Critique (i.e., think through strengths/limitations of the methods and results; address the key questions listed, and add additional comments as needed)
What was the primary outcome of interest?	Is this outcome appropriate for addressing the stated objective?
How was the primary outcome measured? Be specific—include details of measurement tools, assays, etc. used.	Was the measurement of outcome reliable? Was the measurement of outcome valid? What strengths and/or limitations do you note? Could the study results have been affected by **differential** misclassification of outcome? Why or why not? If so, describe direction, magnitude, and likelihood. Could the study results have been affected by **nondifferential** misclassification of the outcome? Why or why not? If so, describe direction, magnitude, and likelihood. Note any additional comments:

5. *Statistical analysis*

Describe (i.e., report just the facts described in the article)	Critique (i.e., think through strengths/limitations of the methods and results; address the key questions listed, and add additional comments as needed)
What statistical analyses were performed?	Is the analytic approach appropriate for testing the specified hypotheses? Why or why not?
How was confounding addressed and controlled? (include both approaches in how the study was designed and how data were analyzed) Describe the important confounders that were considered.	Were these approaches sufficient to control for confounding? What is the likelihood of residual confounding? Should the authors have considered the effect of other variables not included in the study?
What, if any, effect modification was evaluated?	Were the methods to evaluate effect modification sufficient? Why or why not? Note any additional comments:
What is the sample size? (specify total, cases/controls, exposed/unexposed, etc. as appropriate)	Are sample size/power calculations provided? Is there sufficient statistical power for testing the stated hypotheses? Note any additional comments:

6. Results and conclusions

What was the major result of the study? Include information on direction and magnitude of association for most important finding, e.g., give the actual OR and confidence interval, and also interpret the findings in words. Be sure to mention the comparison category in your text (e.g., compared to individuals who did not drink alcohol).

Was the stability of the result assessed (i.e. did the authors report subgroup and/or stratified analyses, explore alternative exposure and/or outcome definitions, etc.?) If so, describe the analyses and their results.

What conclusions do the authors make?

Are these conclusions justified given the results? Why or why not? If not, what conclusions do you feel are appropriate?

How do these findings compare to those of prior studies? What factors might account for any differences noted?

Note any additional comments:

7. Overall assessment

What are the most important strengths of the study? For each, describe in detail why this is an important strength and how it affects internal and/or external validity. Is the potential effect of the strength on the results minor, moderate, or major?

What are the most important limitations of the study? For each, describe in detail why this is an important limitation and how it affects internal and/or external validity? Is the potential effect of the limitation on the results minor, moderate, or major?

How would you characterize the overall quality of the study?

□Poor □Good □Excellent

Justify your choice.

Write a *brief* summary of the article, describing the key methodologic elements, strengths, limitations, and the conclusions that are most appropriate given the article's findings and your assessment of internal validity:

Critical Analysis of Mirick DK, Davis S, and Thomas DB. Antiperspirant use and the risk of breast cancer. *Journal of the National Cancer Institute.* 2002. 94(20): 1578–80

Overview

In this brief article, Mirick et al.[1] report the results of a population-based case-control study evaluating associations between antiperspirant/deodorant use and breast cancer risk. The authors note pervasive rumors circulating in the media and in popular culture that use of underarm antiperspirant or deodorant, especially in combination with shaving the underarm areas, may cause breast cancer, despite a lack of scientific evidence to support such claims. The authors explored these relationships in the context of an ongoing, population-based case-control study. Breast cancer cases (N = 813) aged 20–74 years were identified through a cancer registry in Western Washington State, with controls (N = 793) identified using random-digit dialing from the same source population and frequency-matched to cases in 5-year age groups. Exposure to antiperspirants, deodorants, and underarm shaving was ascertained via in-person interviews. Analysis of the 810 cases and 793 controls with complete exposure data revealed no statistically significant association between ever regularly using antiperspirant (OR 0.9, 95% CI 0.7–1.1) or deodorant (OR 1.2, 95% CI 0.9–1.5) and breast cancer. Similar results were obtained when the antiperspirant or deodorant use was regularly occurring within one hour of shaving (OR 0.9, 95% CI 0.7–1.1; and OR 1.2, 95% CI 0.9–1.5, respectively). Overall, this well-powered study does not support an association between underarm use of antiperspirant or deodorant, with or without coincident shaving, and breast cancer risk. These results are reassuring, in that this common set of behaviors is unlikely to lead to increased breast cancer risk.

Study population

While few details regarding the recruitment of the study participants are provided in this brief article, readers are referred to two earlier publications for complete methodology.[2,3] Eligible cases were White females ages 20–74 who were newly diagnosed with breast cancer between November 1992 and March 1995 and had a telephone in their homes. Eligible cases were identified from a cancer registry covering two counties in Western

Washington State, with sampling done to ensure representation across urban, suburban, and rural areas. Of 1,039 eligible cases, 813 (78%) agreed to participate. Controls identified through random-digit-dialing were eligible if they were female, White, lived in one of the same two counties as cases, and had no personal history of breast cancer. Controls were frequency-matched to cases in 5-year age groups. Of the 1,053 eligible controls, 793 (75%) agreed to participate.

The rigorous recruitment methodology ensured that cases and controls arose from the same source population and were comparable to one another. Eligibility criteria were the same for cases and controls, except with respect to breast cancer diagnosis. There is minimal potential for selection bias given the consistent eligibility criteria and similarly high response rates. While results should be broadly generalizable to White females, the external validity for other racial/ethnic groups is unclear; given known differences in breast cancer risk by race/ethnicity, additional research in racially and ethnically diverse populations is needed. The sample size is large, providing sufficient power (80%) to detect OR = 1.24 as statistically significant with $\alpha = 0.05$.

Exposure assessment

Participants provided information on their exposure to antiperspirants and deodorants through in-person interviews. Based on their responses, investigators were able to evaluate both products categorized as exclusive use (yes/no), ever regular use (yes/no), and regular use within one hour of shaving (yes/no).

Overall, the exposure assessment method has several limitations. First, interviewer bias, in which interviewers question cases and controls differently, may have occurred and is a major concern, especially if interviewers were aware of the rumored link between antiperspirant/deodorant use and breast cancer. Although cases and controls were asked the same questions, the articles did not state that interviewers were masked to participants' disease status,[1-3] thus creating an opportunity for differential misclassification of exposure to occur.

Second, the self-reported nature of the exposure creates opportunities for non-differential misclassification of exposure, as both cases and controls may have difficulty remembering and accurately reporting their exposure to antiperspirant and deodorant. However, given that these behaviors tend to be long-term habits, this is a minor concern.

Third, there also is potential for non-differential misclassification of exposure resulting from the lack of specific information on frequency and duration of product use and also categorizing essentially as ever versus never, which lacks information on use during specific periods of susceptibility that are relevant to future breast cancer risk. It is also possible that participants reported their current use of these products, which may not reflect their use prior to breast cancer diagnosis or a similar historical period for controls. This is a moderate concern.

Fourth, there is a moderate concern that recall bias may have occurred; breast cancer cases may have been searching for explanations for their diagnosis, potentially leading to more or less accurate recall than controls.

While these limitations are substantial and lower internal validity of the study, it is also important to note that self-report is the only possible approach to collecting data on this exposure, which would not be recorded in medical records or other existing documentation.

Outcome assessment

Breast cancer cases were identified via a cancer registry at the Fred Hutchinson Cancer Research Center. Cases diagnosed between November 1992 and March 1995 with International Classification of Diseases for Oncology (ICD-O) codes 174.0–174.9 were selected.[2,3] Overall, this is a highly rigorous approach for identifying incident breast cancer cases, making misclassification of outcome unlikely. The cancer registry covered the two counties that formed the source population for recruitment of cases and controls, ensuring that all residents of these counties with a breast cancer diagnosis were identified.

Because breast cancer diagnosis would be made without knowledge of underarm hygiene habits, differential misclassification of outcome is not a concern. However, there is a minor concern that non-differential misclassification of outcomes could have occurred. Because some breast cancer cases are diagnosed based solely on mammographic findings, it is possible that some controls may have undetected breast cancer, although this is only a minor concern. The authors did not describe how controls were verified not to have a personal diagnosis of breast cancer.[2,3]

Statistical analysis

Multivariable-adjusted odds ratios and 95% confidence intervals were calculated using conditional logistic regression models. This is an appropriate analytic approach given the matched case-control study design. These models were adjusted for age, parity, age at first pregnancy, first-degree female relative with breast cancer, double oophorectomy before age 40, oral contraceptive use, history of upper gastrointestinal x-ray, smoking history, mother/sister with breast cancer before age 45, alcohol consumption (if premenopausal), and hormone therapy use (if postmenopausal). While this is a comprehensive set of confounders, there was no adjustment for other potential confounders (e.g., body mass index, physical activity), leaving a minor to moderate concern for residual confounding. Also, there is no explanation provided for adjusting for history of upper gastrointestinal x-ray. Because this medical procedure is not linked to breast cancer diagnosis nor associated with underarm hygiene, it is unlikely to confound the exposure-outcome relationship under study and may represent an overadjustment.

Effect modification was not assessed, although menopausal status is known to modify associations between other exposures (e.g., obesity) and breast cancer risk.

Finally, the study had sufficient statistical power for evaluating the tested hypotheses, as described earlier. Although the authors did not report their available statistical power, calculations based on their reported data revealed 80% power to detect a relatively small OR of 1.24 with two-sided $\alpha = 0.05$.

Overall assessment

Mirick et al.[1] provide compelling evidence that underarm use of antiperspirants or deodorant is not related to breast cancer risk. While the study does have some important limitations, especially related to exposure assessment, the strengths far outweigh the limitations. Overall, this study was of good quality, and the authors provide an appropriate interpretation of their findings, which do not support causal links between antiperspirant or deodorant use and breast cancer risk.

The study is significantly strengthened by its rigorous recruitment methodology and outcome assessment. Importantly, cases and controls were selected from the same source population, had similarly high participation rates, and met similar eligibility criteria, limiting the potential for selection bias. Incident breast cancer outcomes were identified through a cancer registry, which is a highly valid approach and minimized differential and non-differential misclassification of the outcome. Furthermore, the rigorous statistical analysis utilized an appropriate analytic approach, adjusted for important confounders, and was well-powered for testing the study hypotheses.

There are, however, several limitations. Most importantly, the exposure assessment has a high potential for differential misclassification as a result of possible interviewer bias and recall bias given the case-control design and the failure to mask interviewers to disease status. Differential misclassification of antiperspirant and/or deodorant use would most likely bias results away from the null hypothesis and lead to an apparent positive association between these exposures and breast cancer. Given that positive associations were not observed; however, we are reassured that any impact of differential misclassification was minimal. Non-differential misclassification is also a potential concern, given that exposure status was self-reported and only classified as ever versus never. This measurement error would tend to bias results toward the null hypothesis and may explain the reported lack of association. Finally, the study participants all identified as White, and results may not be generalizable to females of other races and ethnicities given known differences in breast cancer risk by race/ethnicity.

Overall, this study supports a conclusion that underarm use of antiperspirants and deodorant, with or without shaving, is not associated with breast cancer risk. Future studies that utilize a more rigorous exposure assessment approach and recruit a racially and ethnically diverse study population will be important for confirming these findings. However, this rigorous study that observed no association should offer reassurance to females that these behaviors are unlikely to impact their future risk of breast cancer.

References

1. Mirick DK, Davis S, Thomas DB. Antiperspirant use and the risk of breast cancer. *J Natl Cancer Inst.* 2002;94(20):1578–1580. doi:10.1093/jnci/94.20.1578
2. Davis S, Mirick DK, Stevens RG. Night shift work, light at night, and risk of breast cancer. *J Natl Cancer Inst.* 2001;93(20):1557–1562. doi:10.1093/jnci/93.20.1557
3. Davis S, Mirick DK, Stevens RG. Residential magnetic fields and the risk of breast cancer. *Am J Epidemiol.* 2002;155(5):446–454. doi:10.1093/aje/155.5.446

Index

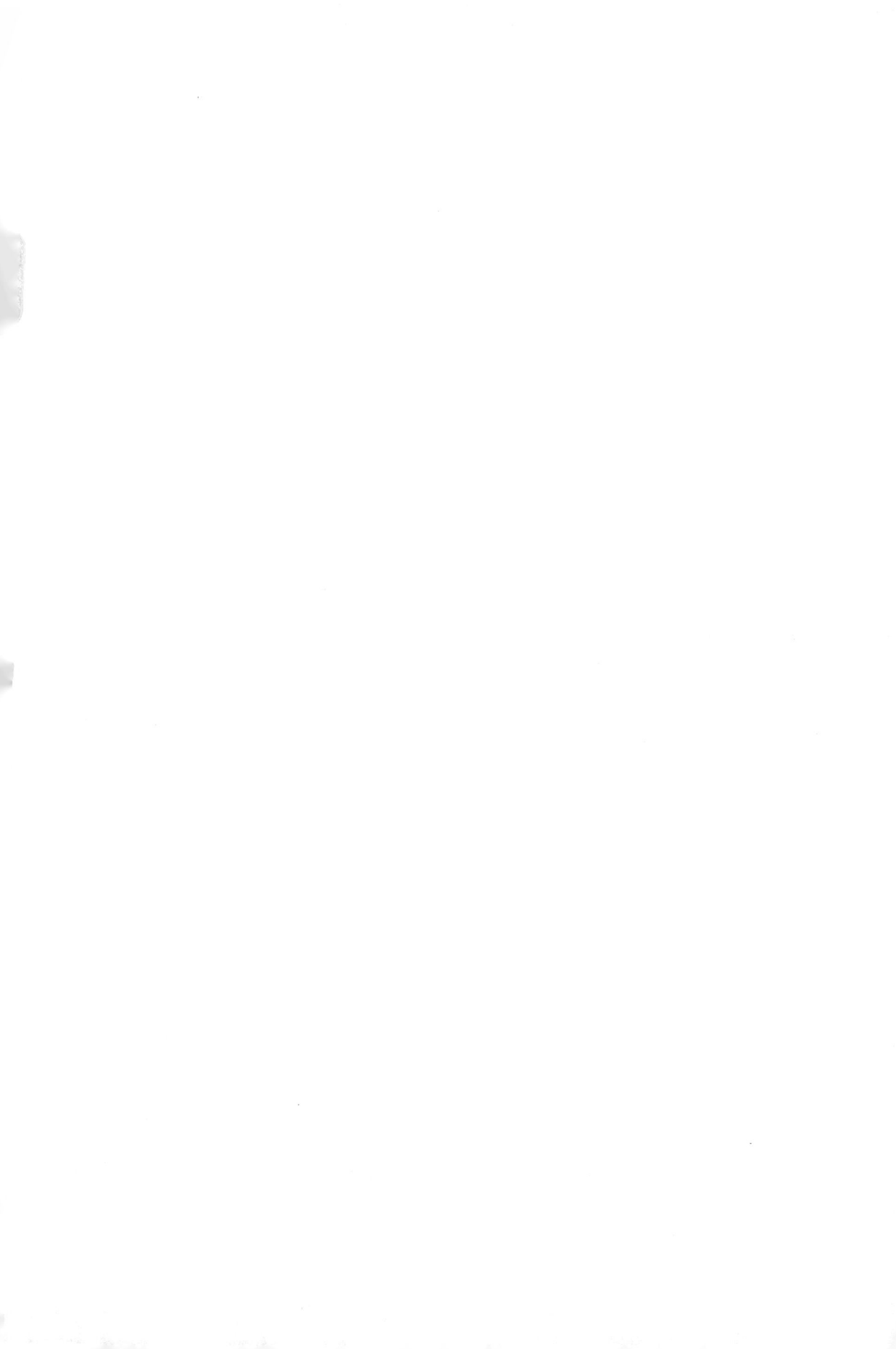

For Product Safety Concerns and Information please contact our EU
representative GPSR@taylorandfrancis.com
Taylor & Francis Verlag GmbH, Kaufingerstraße 24, 80331 München, Germany

www.ingramcontent.com/pod-product-compliance
Lightning Source LLC
Chambersburg PA
CBHW081106220326
41598CB00038B/7244

* 9 7 8 1 0 4 1 0 6 9 2 5 6 *